CW00665118

© **Copyright 2020 - All rights reserved.**

The content contained within this book may not be reproduced, duplicated or transmitted without direct written permission from the author or the publisher.

Under no circumstances will any blame or legal responsibility be held against the publisher, or author, for any damages, reparation, or monetary loss due to the information contained within this book, either directly or indirectly.

Legal Notice:

This book is copyright protected. It is only for personal use. You cannot amend, distribute, sell, use, quote or paraphrase any part, or the content within this book, without the consent of the author or publisher.

Disclaimer Notice:

Please note the information contained within this document is for educational and entertainment purposes only. All effort has been executed to present accurate, up to date, reliable, complete information. No warranties of any kind are declared or implied. Readers acknowledge that the author is not engaged in the rendering of legal, financial, medical or professional advice. The content within this book has been derived from various sources. Please consult a licensed professional before attempting any techniques outlined in this book.

By reading this document, the reader agrees that under no circumstances is the author responsible for any losses, direct or indirect, that are incurred as a result of the use of the information contained within this document, including, but not limited to, errors, omissions, or inaccuracies.

Table of Contents

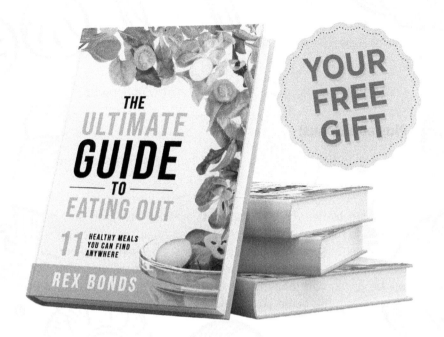

Before we get started, I'd like to offer you this free gift. It's my way of saying thank you for spending time with me in this book. Your gift is a Special Report titled, **"The Ultimate Guide To Eating Out: 11 Healthy Meals You Can Find Anywhere."** It's an easy-to-use guide that pulls together a ton of analysis I've previously only shared with clients. I think you're going to love it. This guide is a collection of 11 Healthy Meals you can find anywhere that will give you the system, tools, info, and mindset you need on the path to achieving your fitness dreams. This guide will teach you where to find clean, nutrition-packed meals to build lean muscle, burn fat and bump up your confidence in every situation no matter where you are.

Scan Me
To Claim Your Free Gift!

In this guide you'll learn:

✓ Where to find the 11 healthiest meals when you're eating out

✓ A rock-solid meal plan for any time of day & every location

✓ The exact script for which menu items to order

✓ Nutritional information for each dish at your fingertips

Plus as a Bonus!

✓ A Nutrition and fitness Journal to stay on track daily to your fitness dreams!

I'm willing to bet you'll find at least a few ideas, tools and meals covered in that guide that will surprise and help you. This guide will set you up for success and is a proven system when eating out. With this guide you will be armed with the info & focus you need. You will be giving your body nutritious fuel and enjoy eating out. With downloading this guide, you're taking a solid step on the path to your fitness success.

How can you obtain a copy of *The Ultimate Guide To Eating Out: 11 Healthy Meals You Can Find Anywhere?* It's simple. Visit RexBondsBooks.com and sign up for my email list (or simply click the link above). You'll receive immediate access to the Report in PDF format. You can read it online, download it or print it out. You will also get a Free Fitness Journal and Planner for signing up for my email list as well. Everything you need to get started and stay on your fitness journey is included in **signing up for my email list.**

Being on my email list also means you'll be the first to know when I release a new health and fitness book. I plan to release my books at a steep discount (or even free) for the first 24 hours. By signing up for my email list you'll get an early notification.

If you don't want to join my list, that's completely fine. This just means I need to earn your trust. With this in mind, I think you are going to love the information I've included in the ultimate guide. More specifically, I think you're going to love what it can do for your life.

Without further ado, let's jump into this book.

Join the Rex Bonds Fitness Community

Looking to build your specific fitness habits and goals? If so, then check out the Rex Bonds Fitness community: Rex Bonds Fitness Group

This is an amazing group full of like-minded individuals who focus on getting results with their lives. Here you can discover simple strategies, build powerful habits, find accountability partners and ask questions about your struggles. If you want to "level up" in your fitness journey, then this is the place to be.

**Just scan the QR code below
to join the Rex Bonds Fitness Community.**

Introduction

Do you have bloating, digestion, anxiety, and weight problems? Perhaps you even spent countless hours researching books, videos, and websites and came to the conclusion, "I think my problem might have to do with my gut."

I'm here to tell you that yes... it could be your gut, but right now, it is not 100% scientifically proven that healing your gut is linked to reducing bloating, digestion, anxiety, and fat loss problems. There are so many more factors involved in these diseases that aren't entirely determined by your gut, and there's so much we still need to learn about the microbiome. Despite this fact, there are so many people out there taking advantage of the progress we're making in the field of gut health by promoting their product, service, or FAD diet to make people think, "Maybe if I fix my gut, then I can fix my bloating, digestion, anxiety and lose weight." In this book, I will be going over the truth on what is scientifically proven on how gut health correlates to bloating, digestion, mental health, and fat loss.

As a fitness guide, nutrition coach, author, and certified health and wellness instructor, I have trained hundreds of people. A majority of my clients always wanted to talk to me about their gut health, and at the time, I wanted to know more about this topic, as well. It sounded like heaven to my clients that "healing my gut is what I have been missing out on my whole life!" So I dove into countless hours of testing methods and went over tons and tons of scientific articles to find the answer. Answers I feel my clients deserved to have since they truly do mean the world to me. I wanted my clients to have the most accurate information and the best results possible. My search for truth has brought me back to where I started. It seems the more things change, the more they remain the same. Often, the answers we're all looking for are hidden in plain sight. I wanted to give my clients the results they wanted, the practical tools for their success, and a no-nonsense blueprint they can follow. This is my mission with every book I write, to make sure you achieve the body you deserve.

After tireless research and testing, I have been able to discern myths from facts and everything in between. Through my efforts, my clients have now gained the knowledge they need to sift through all these new products, fad diets, and people claiming to heal your gut and help them make the right choices for their health. My clients are now saving their precious time, money, and health from many of these companies and products that are claiming to heal their gut.

My clients thank me now for how much clarity this information has brought them, because it is so hard to know what information is true in this day and age, especially regarding our gut health. Before, they were confused about what to believe. This book really opened their eyes and allowed them to see what the scientific and clinical consensus is right now. The unbiased approach is what is most appreciated about my work.

In this book, I promise you will understand 100% on how your gut correlates to your bloating, digestion, anxiety, and fat loss problem. I will be sourcing real reputable, scientifically reviewed journals while presenting you the information in the most accessible way possible. You will gain the knowledge you need to further assist you in your healing journey, and sift through all this misinformation about how your gut health correlates to bloating, digestion, anxiety, and fat loss. I even hired a professional medical writer to make sure everything in this book is backed up by real science.

I will also show you what science has to say about the right and proven methods that exist, which can help you deal with anxiety, obesity, inflammation, and gut health. You will come to see that there is really no cutting corners when it comes to your wellbeing. There is much work to be done, but the first step in the process is awareness. Once you become aware of how you can begin to heal yourself, you will then need the insight and tools to carry on with the process. This is where my practical advice comes in, and I'm going to give you the tools necessary to begin to create change in your life because awareness without insight leaves you with nothing more than frustration.

As we go on this journey of discovery and scrutiny, you'll come to see that things aren't as simple as mainstream media would have you believe. Our gut is not an isolated system. It's part of a whole, just like we're part of a whole. As Aristotle once illustrated, the whole is larger than the sum of its parts. The interactions between our gut, the rest of our body, and our social-economic system are what we're going to learn to take into account. We must look at the whole picture, and this is what the term "health" implies anyway.

At the end of the day, I want the best possible solution for you. Solutions that anybody can and should incorporate into their lifestyles. I want you to make informed decisions for your body and health but specifically your gut health. So, the faster you act, the faster your health, body, and gut are going to thank you in the long run. As a little reminder, this is ongoing work, and there is much of it to be done.

This book is backed by 100% real published works by reputable scientific research sites such as Nature. This information will help you understand where the scientific debate stands regarding gut health and what is actually known about our body. Each chapter in this book will provide you with up to date, 100% real, reputable, scientifically reviewed studies on gut health and its relationships to bloating, digestion, mental health, and fat loss. After reading this book, you shouldn't have to ever go on another extreme fad diet, take all these new expensive supplements, or pay an arm and a leg to a person that claims they can heal your gut.

CHAPTER 01
HISTORY OF GUT HEALTH

In this chapter, I would like to help you look at the big picture and understand why and how we have turned our attention towards our gut.

First, we'll talk about our relationship to disease and the different conceptions we've had about it throughout history.

Along with our conception of disease, we also need to take a look at the aspects of our lives that have drastically changed in recent years with the advancement of technology and civilization.

Then we must question the information that is being tossed around as scientific truth by reviewing recent developments in the field of microbiology and genetics.

The War Against Unseen Forces

We may begin to understand humankind's conception of illness and disease by looking at the words themselves. The term "disease" or "disease" refers to the unease, discomfort, and pain you would feel when ill (Cohen, 1953). On the other hand, the word "health" refers to the idea of being whole. It may be that our ancestors looked at being unhealthy, like missing out on some aspect of life or not having enough of something. This may be what was implied by not being whole, by being fragmented as a system or being in a state of disharmony.

Our more primitive ancestors cared much more about the cure than the origin of a disease. This preoccupation with the cure, without addressing the root cause, led them to superstitious and magical practices as a means for a cure (Cohen, 1953). As we well know, some of the more esoteric practices may have really worked—they may have treated the symptoms—but they didn't know exactly what it was about the rituals that cured the person. This tendency to apply cures without understanding the underlying mechanisms is dangerous and misleading; this tendency still occurs in our current era.

We have given different explanations as to why ill fate befalls us, why people become sick, or why some are simply born different. Some schools of thought would blame a sinful lifestyle for plagues and epidemics. In those times, religion, philosophy, and medicine were all a single discipline, which led to one of the most primitive conceptions of disease; the idea that disease was caused by a demonic entity. Evil spirits were thought to enter the body, and then they would look to reproduce and propagate. Treatment ranged from carrying a new potato in your pocket to an exorcism (Cohen, 1953).

Jumping ahead to the eighteenth century, an idea of disease as a deviation from normality or a disruption in equilibrium was born from Greek thought (Cohen, 1953). These ideas match fairly well with our current conceptions of wellbeing. Particularly, the idea of homeostasis that refers to the dynamic harmonious state in a self-sustaining biological system.

One last theory that was held in more recent years is that of miasma; as you will see, this concept is extremely relevant and still influences the public's outlook on gut health. The most recent definition of miasma is the "harmful air produced by nature." Miasma was an ancient idea that stuck with us up until the nineteenth century. This pestilent air was thought to come from swamps and forests mainly; it was considered to be the cause of disease for quite some time (Shumsky, N., 1998). In other words, miasma was looked at as air that contained harmful properties for humans. The underlying unconscious belief was that nature could be toxic for humans.

The next assumption we made after miasma was that, if nature was the culprit behind diseases, then man-made chemicals must be clean. We should be able to cleanse our cities through the use of chemicals by eliminating any pestilence originating from nature.

Keep this idea of artificial chemicals being the source of purity and cleanliness in your mind as we continue to move forward into our modern era.

In the nineteenth century, we found a new enemy to rage war against: germs. As the concept of germs rose in popularity, most began to discard the idea of miasma. Germs were the new culprits for disease. The war on germs was directly related to an increase in our standards of hygiene. Fluoride and chlorine were introduced into our water streams, and deaths associated with cholera infections practically disappeared.

Antibiotics were then the next step in our attempt to destroy pathogenic bacteria, and we truly did succeed for the most part. Hygiene and antibiotics have contributed to an increase in our life expectancy (Bloomfield, Smith, & Rook, 2012).

For the longest time, we had blamed unseen forces for our diseases. Now we know that there truly are unseeable forces at work. Unseeable to the naked eye at least.

Our gut is inhabited by trillions of microorganisms, making up our microbial ecosystem. This ecosystem is vital to our metabolic energy-producing processes. Pharmaceutical alcohol, chlorine, and antibiotics were all designed to kill microorganisms. At what cost did we win the war against germs?

There is an idea called the hygiene hypothesis. This idea blames our modern lifestyle and our increased levels of hygiene for the increase in allergic and autoimmune diseases such as arthritis, asthma, and food allergies (Smith, Bloomfield, & Rook, 2012). It states that we were far too successful in our endeavors against germs and that we've been destroying a lot of our good bacteria along with the pathogens. Now you would imagine that these sorts of diseases would decrease instead of increase with our standards of cleanliness and the advancement of medicine, right?

It's understandable why the hygiene hypothesis has become so popular. There are large amounts of studies on germ-free mice (GFM) that show just how important it is for a mammal to have a prosperous microbial ecosystem. GFM are mice that have been isolated from microbes; therefore, they never had the chance to be colonized; in other words, they're sterile. It has been noticed that GFM display learning and memory deficits as compared to specific pathogen-free mice (SPFM) (Clarke et al., 2013; Gareau et al., 2011; Heijtz et al., 2011; Neufeld et al., 2011 as cited in Sharon et. al., 2016). This is one of the many detrimental effects caused by having few to no microorganisms in their gut.

The hygiene hypothesis proposes that one of the reasons allergies are on the rise is because of a lack of exposure to good bacteria, which makes it so we are not appropriately colonized. Perhaps you have met somebody who would not allow their child to play with dirt or who would not allow pets in the house because they see them as germ producing factories. Could they be doing their child more harm than good by being overprotective and not allowing them to increase their microbial biodiversity through colonization? More than likely, yes.

A statistically relevant study (Schmidt et al., as cited in Benede et. al., 2016) shows that children who have pets or older siblings are less likely to develop food allergies.

Schmidt (as cited in Bened et. al., 2016) then tested his theory on piglets, as well, and the results were positive there too. Another study on GFM showed that brushing pet dust on the mice served as a protective measure against asthma (Fujimura et. al., as cited in Benede et. al., 2016). The results from these studies seem to draw a relationship between our exposure to bacteria throughout our development and the manifestation of certain autoimmune diseases.

In regards to the part about having older siblings, the hygiene hypothesis also takes into consideration the fact that family sizes in developed countries have decreased (Smith, Bloomfield, & Rook, 2012). This can account for the decreased exposure to good bacteria that is proposed, which is necessary to have a thriving microbial ecosystem in our gut. We exchange bacteria with our siblings through various means, mainly orally through saliva. We will talk about colonization in great detail in the following chapter.

These studies truly make us rethink our relationship with "germs" and makes us wonder if we have demonized them too much. Perhaps we should stop seeing things in black and white, as all good or all bad. There's a lot of gray area in between, a lot of space that allows for scrutiny and analysis.

From Delusions to Fads

Another old idea has made its way into modern thought. There has always been a certain resistance to science and scrutiny. Perhaps it's because, with science, there is room for the unknown and uncertainty. The idea that has crept its way into modern society is that of an antagonism between food and medicine.

"Let food be thy medicine and medicine be thy food," Some people have tried to use this quote, attributed to Hippocrates, to transmit that we have strayed away from a more natural path of wellbeing. That since ancient times, the Greeks knew that food was a superior alternative to medicine. Perhaps it may be a type of neophobia (fear of the new) that makes people reject all those things that are artificial or synthetic.

Many gut health enthusiasts may have you believe that microbial supplements and more "natural" alternatives are far superior to the methods practiced by the medical establishment.

Interestingly, the quote that I previously provided you is that research shows that Hippocrates never did say that. It is just something people started saying he said to further the credibility of their own ideas (Cardenas, 2013).

We must stop seeing things in black and white terms. We can't go around discarding natural alternatives and ancient knowledge or seeing scientific breakthroughs as conspiracies that have been put in place to control us. We have the anti-vaccine people trying to bring chickenpox back, for example, which goes quite well with the hygiene hypothesis; it's a rejection of civilization. Now, I'm sure that to some extent, pharmaceutical companies should be less profit-oriented and more solution-centered. There's a little bit of truth to both sides of the argument, and science can help us arrive at some sort of a middle ground.

Nutrition is definitely among the best preventive measures against diseases. I am by no means devaluing alternative and natural approaches to health. All I am asking of you is to have a healthy level of skepticism. Have enough faith and humility to allow yourself to know that there are things you don't know, but at the same time, don't be blinded by faith alone.

The internet and social media have changed the way many of us consume information. When it comes to gut health, you have to be able to discern whether or not people truly have your best interest at heart, or if they're just trying to make a buck off of a new fad. It's terrible because what they're selling you is hope. Even if their intent isn't ill, what are their qualifications? Why do they have a solution while hundreds of scientists are still struggling to find an answer? Are they merely cherry-picking studies while ignoring the ones that contradict their ideas?

The field of gut health is currently booming with 12,900 publications in the last 7 years (Cani, 2018). Those publications make up 80% of all the publications on the topic in the last 40 years. Like I said, it's mainly due to technological advancements, but there is, understandably, a lot of excitement around the topic. I just want you to think twice before you hop on the hype train.

People will see what they want to see; a person can look at the research in a biased fashion and distort the results to meet their ends. Sure, there are a ton of correlations being found, but we have not yet found a sure way to apply the knowledge we have come across.

There is no failproof way to manipulate the microbial ecosystem in your gut, YET. This is the fact to this day. People in the field of gut health should be cautious not to make false promises. I'm going to help you look at actual facts so you can make up your own mind about the matter at hand.

Now, I will address the reasons for which you're interested in gut health and help you on your healing journey.

Dysbiosis: The New Culprit

A constant war is being waged in our gut; parasitic organisms including fungi, archaea, and bacteria against the commensal beings that aid our metabolic processes. What determines which side wins the war though? The side that wins the war is the side you feed.

Could there be things we do to sabotage our commensal microorganisms?

With the knowledge about this war in our gut, the public has become increasingly aware of the importance of beneficial bacteria, to the point that some people have started to devalue our standards of hygiene, which can be dangerous. Needless to say, we should be very grateful for the changes that have taken place in regards to our hygienic practices.

One aspect of our hygienic practices people are growing increasingly uncomfortable with is the excessive use of antibiotics. Antibiotic residues in animals also prove to be a cause for concern. We administer antibiotics to our livestock, so they survive the conditions that we keep them in without becoming infected by pathogenic bacteria. This relates to us because we can then consume the residues from antibiotics given to our livestock in dairy and meat, which may destroy the good bacteria in our gut along with the bad. After all, that is what antibiotics are designed to do.

Experiments administering antibiotics to mice have been successful in flushing a large amount of the biodiversity out of their gut (Savage & Johns as cited in, Benede et. al., 2016). Interestingly, after the mice's microbial ecosystem had been destroyed by excessive antibiotics, they began to develop an allergy to peanuts. An allergy born from an overly sensitive immune system. We'll discuss the relationship between our microbial ecosystem and the development of our immune system at a later time.

Dysbiosis in our gut refers to an imbalance in our microbial flora. This is thought to occur by not having a big enough micro-biodiversity and allowing specific strains of microorganisms to overpopulate our gut. Biodiversity is believed to be diminished by smaller family sizes, chlorine, and fluoride in the water, antibiotics in our food, and antibiotics as means to treat microbial infections, along with chronically increased stress levels.

These are all possibilities and ideas that deserve to be explored, and they are being investigated. Correlations are being found, and evidence to support the hypotheses is being proposed. These are exciting times to be alive, and a lot of scientific and clinical breakthroughs are still occurring, but there's also much to be learned. The fact that there's much to be learned is what motivates researchers to study this topic more. The more mystery there is around a subject, the more discoveries are to be made. At the same time, the high amount of research being done in the field is indicative of how little we truly know about the subject.

Perhaps what we should have learned from our story of attempting to find culprits for disease is that we should really look to treat the root cause. Identify the root cause before we start treating symptoms, and maybe that there isn't just one single culprit, but an array of factors that interplay with each other.

I'm sure that proponents of miasma or demonic possessions as causes for illness adamantly believed they had found an ultimate truth that should be shared with all humanity. They must have really felt like they were doing people a service.

On the other hand, I'm positive there were charlatans who simply took advantage of people's need to point the finger at a culprit. People need to feel safe, a safety brought through promises of longevity and wellbeing. Humans don't seem to like uncertainty, so giving people a target to blame can be a great way to befriend folks. This appears to be happening with our microbial ecosystem. People are taking advantage and cherry-picking studies and evidence to fit their own needs.

The only difference between the people who wanted to help mankind and the charlatans who took advantage of the ignorance of others is the intention with which they carried themselves. In both cases, they were misinforming people, and possibly doing them more harm than good.

We have come a long way since blaming ethereal entities for our illnesses. Just like in the past, in present times, there are also people who think they have found the ultimate truth, that they have finally discovered our culprits for disease. In our current era, our culprit is gut dysbiosis. People have come to the idea that gut dysbiosis is the cause for many of our modern era's diseases, namely depression, obesity, anxiety, gastrointestinal issues, hormonal imbalances, and autoimmune diseases. As we'll come to see, dysbiosis is but one factor in play. It's an important factor, but it's not an isolated system because it interacts with many other systems.

There is still a large amount of debate about how we should research and analyze the microbes in our gut, but one thing is for sure. Stool samples have been used quite a lot in recent years, but we now know that there are microorganisms that can't be studied in stool. Many of the microbes that are mucosally adherent and those that reside in the small intestine don't show up in your stool (Allaband et. al., 2019). Another limitation of stool research is that it's challenging to determine where the

The Secrets To Improve Bloating, Digestion, Anxiety And Fat Loss

bacteria they find are coming from. Is it the small intestine, colon, stomach, liver?

Stool has proven to be useful in many cases where pathology was present, but we're not able to see the whole picture through these studies.

In order for you to get a good idea of the myths that we have progressed from recently, let's take the slogan many gut health enthusiasts still use; some people would use the statement that we have 10 times the amount of microorganisms than we do cells in our body. Now, we know that this isn't the case. However, people still use this outdated fact to make the microbiome seem more important than all the other processes in your body and mind. They would have us believe that if you have more microbes than you do cells in your body, then you should probably be paying just as much or more attention to your microbiome as you do the rest of your body. Therefore, it is imperative that you buy their product in order to heal your gut; that's the kind of discourse that is being used.

We now know that the truth is closer to a 1:1 ratio rather than a 10:1 ratio. This wouldn't sound quite as good as having ten times the amount of microbes in your body as you do cells though (Allaband et. al., 2019). This shift in our body's constitution shows just how much we've learned and how much we didn't know about the human body in recent years.

Our knowledge about our microbiome drastically changed in 2007, when the Human Microbiome Project (HMP) began. This was an international effort to study the microbiome. The reason it was so successful is because this was when we really started to incorporate genome sequencing into our methods with which we study our microorganisms (Rogers, 2016). Only within the first three years of the HMP, we discovered 200 new species of microorganisms. It's safe to say that you should be wary of any research done prior to 2007, since our knowledge about the microbiome was fairly limited then.

The idea behind dysbiosis is that there are commensal bacteria and other less beneficial pathogens. Commensal bacteria are organisms that we share a symbiotic relationship with, meaning that we benefit from coexisting with them as much as they benefit from us. Commensal bacteria don't necessarily have to benefit us, but they must simply not hinder our wellbeing.

Lactobacillus and Bifidobacterium are some of the more popular strains supported by gut health enthusiasts; they are supposed to be the good guys. The idea that is being tossed around as truth is that having more of these strains in your gut will lead to better health.

Pathogens are organisms that have more parasitic relationships with us. They're much like that freeloading friend that is always mooching off of you without so much as a thank you. They're only in it for themselves; their survival and progress come at the cost of our wellbeing. Candida Albicans is a strain of fungi that inhabits our gut and has been targeted as a pathogen. Excessive amounts of this pathogen is thought to cause intestinal wall permeability or leaky gut (Zuo & Siew, 2018).

I will demystify some of these ideas, and discuss the reasons why people have jumped to conclusions. We'll be reviewing the mechanisms from where the assumptions about commensal and pathogenic bacteria have been born.

It's challenging to pinpoint a single microorganism and blame it for a specific disease (Cani, 2018). There are other factors that should be considered since no research shows that a single strain is responsible for obesity. It may be the chemicals our microorganisms produce, it could be the quality or quantity of those chemicals, or it may be our own cell's sensitivity to these chemicals that are the causes.

These are promising future areas for study. We will view the most recent findings to make sure we're up to date with the current state of the debates surrounding our microbiome.

In the literature regarding gut health, correlations are often drawn between a specific organism and a disease. Correlations are drawn without really knowing what the underlying mechanisms are. Now, it's not like researchers are lazy, and they don't want to look into it; It's more due to how difficult and time consuming it is to study such a complex system (Cani, 2018)

If you were to make a claim that states the higher the amount of Lactobacillus you have, the healthier your gut will be, you then have to go on to prove this fact. This is one of the ideas backing up a lot of probiotic products. One way you can prove an idea, such as the one previously stated, is by isolating the organism and making sure that it's actually this organism that is responsible for our microbial equilibrium.

Isolating an organism of this sort comes with its challenges. Even when researchers are able to culture an appropriate quantity of the targeted organism, the data that is born from such studies has its limitations. These organisms aren't isolated in our gut; they're part of a whole system. There are many other bacterial colonies and cells that these organisms interact with. We can't study an isolated organism and jump to conclusions about its role in disease without testing it in the interconnected system it resides in (Cani, 2018).

Unfortunately, results have not been conclusive to support the idea that having more of a single type of good bacteria helps your microbiome stay healthy (Cani, 2018). The consensus is leaning more towards the idea that having a more diverse microbiome, in general, is the factor related to better health.

We're coming to understand that a single strain of microbes does not have a single function (Cani, 2018). Just like us, these organisms have learned to adapt to their environment. Commensal bacteria can turn into pathogenic bacteria depending on the type of diet you have, and the kinds of bacteria that have colonized you throughout your life.

In this same sense, your microbiome is ever-changing. The things you eat, your stress levels, and the exposure you have to microorganisms may all cause changes in the constitution of your microbial ecosystem. My point is that things are a bit more complex than people would have us believe. I understand that the findings are fascinating and promising, the future looks good, but we must question what a person's intention is when they bypass scientific scrutiny. We must be humble enough to question ourselves and accept the fact that things may be a little more complicated than we think.

So what DO we know? Microbes have different functions depending on the lifestyle we live and what organisms colonized us. Having a diverse ecosystem in our gut is what seems to best correlate with a healthy gut. We should be paying closer attention to more recent studies since the way we study the microbiome, and what we know about it has changed drastically since 2007.

In the following chapter, I'll be able to dive deeper into what we know about the microbiome. Understanding the microbiome's constitution will help you discern information you receive from different media sources a lot better.

CHAPTER 02
MICROBIOME VS. MICROBIOTA

We're going to get into the intricacies that make up the field of gut health. I'm going to be giving you the knowledge required for you to be able to understand any literature you come across about the microbiome. It's your responsibility to read through this chapter carefully. First, we'll define the term gut to better understand the terms microbiome, microbiota, and dysbiosis.

The "Gut"

We've been using the term "gut" loosely throughout this book without really explaining what is meant by it. You may have a vague idea about what the term may mean, but let's define it. The term "gut" refers to the section in our gastrointestinal tract between our stomach's pyloric sphincter and our anus. To be clear, our stomach is not included within the term gut. However, this isn't to say that other organs, like our stomach, liver, and pancreas don't influence the guts functions.

The gut itself is divided into two sections, the small intestine or small bowel and the large intestine or colon. The small intestine is further divided into three sections; the section that meets your pyloric sphincter is called the duodenum. The section in the middle is the jejunum, and the section that reaches your colon is the ileum.

The small intestine is where a large part of our digestion occurs. The digestive process begins when we put food in our mouth, but for now, let's skip to when it gets to your stomach. In your stomach, the food you eat is mixed with digestive juices which vary in acidity or PH levels. Our stomach acid's PH levels rely on microbial equilibrium. It's known that having too many Helicobacter Pylori or H. Pylori will cause your stomach's PH to decrease (Massarrat, 2016).

The Secrets To Improve Bloating, Digestion, Anxiety And Fat Loss

Once your stomach churns the food you have put in it, it then begins to slowly transfer its contents into the small intestine's duodenum. Once in the small intestine, chyme gets mixed with digestive juices coming from our pancreas, liver, and the small intestine itself.

Digestion now takes place—the breaking down or separation of complex molecules into simpler ones. We can either break molecules down mechanically or enzymatically (Ebneshsahidi, 2006). The molecules are then broken down or digested so we can efficiently absorb them into our bloodstream and transport them to the rest of our body.

Absorption in the duodenum takes place through the implementation of finger-like protrusions. They're like little fingers reaching out from the walls of our small intestines with even smaller fingers on them. The large set of fingers are called villi, and the villi have microvilli on them. An image is worth more than a hundred words in this case.

lumen of small intestine

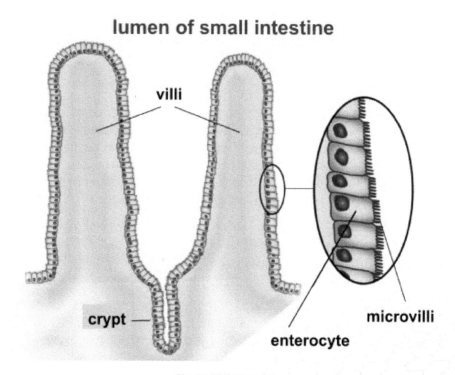

Fig. 1: Villi & Microvilli

As you can see, the image also references the 'lumen' of the small intestine. The lumen is what the intestinal wall is called. One can notice how ingenious nature is by creating such protrusions. The reason they're designed this way is to cover as much area as possible, enabling our intestinal walls to capture and absorb nutrients efficiently.

The microvilli or brush border, as they're popularly known, are like outwards pouches or sacs. They have enzymes attached to them that serve as catalysts to bring nutrients into our enterocytes (absorptive intestinal cells). Once the molecules are broken down and enter our enterocyte, they are then digested by our cells, and the products are released into our bloodstream (Ebneshsahidi, 2006). This transfer of simple molecules into the bloodstream is what is referred to as absorption.

Each enzyme targets a specific molecule; for example, lactase is an enzymatic protein that splits lactose into galactose and glucose.

While the majority of the digestive processes occur in the duodenum, absorption takes place mainly in the jejunum and ileum.

At the end of the ileum, we come across the colon or the large intestine. The colon is characterized by its increased population of microorganisms. There are microorganisms in the small intestine and the stomach, as we have discussed, but the amount present in the colon is far greater (Ebneshsahidi, 2006).

The waste products or the molecules that weren't properly digested, therefore not absorbed, end up in the colon. Once there, the microorganisms in our colon aid us in digesting whatever waste products are left. Let's keep in mind that the waste they metabolize could, in some situations, be toxic to us, so these organisms are truly doing us a service.

Let's think about lactose intolerance for a second. This condition is derived from a lactase deficiency, meaning that we stop producing the same amount of lactase enzymes as we grow older, at least most of us do. Some people manage to keep their lactase enzymes even into adulthood; this has been happening as an adaptation to the domestication of dairy cows (Misselwitz, Butter, and Verbeke, 2019). Since lactose intolerant individuals are unable to break down lactose in the small intestine, it travels in its complex form all the way to the colon. In the colon, it's digested by the organisms that reside there. These organisms take the lactose and process it themselves, producing gases that cause the bloating and cramping that characterizes this food intolerance.

The bacteria in our colon are there to help us. Normally, they break down the waste we couldn't digest and create products that are quite beneficial to us. These compounds that are born from our waste through a digestive process in the microbiota located in our colon are called metabolites. The most popular metabolites are the short-chained fatty acids (SCFA) called propionate, butyrate, and acetate. Keep these in mind as we move forward in our work since they have been shown to possess essential roles in our wellbeing.

The Microbiota & The Microbiome

The population of microorganisms we have been discussing is referred to as the microbiota. The term "microbiota" refers to systems of commensal, symbiotic, or pathogenic organisms that reside within a specific location or organism. In our case, we're talking about the microbiota that resides in the small and large intestine.

Microbiota in our gut may include fungi, bacteria, archaea, yeasts, and viruses.

On the other hand, the term microbiome encompasses the systems of microorganisms, all their genetic material, and even their products (metabolites). In other words, it's the whole ecosystem of microorganisms in our digestive tract.

Now, we're well aware that these organisms reside within us, but how did they get there? Up until recently, it was thought that we were colonized at birth. We believed that an infant's first interaction with microorganisms occurred when the child would open its mouth and become exposed to the mucousy fluids found in the vaginal canal. Now there's an ongoing debate since we have found small amounts of bacteria within the placenta (Dunn et. al., 2017).

One strain of bacteria found in the vagina is the Lactobacillus genus. This strain seems to ward off certain pathogens by creating metabolites that increase the acidity in the environment, making it inhospitable for pathogens (Dunn et. al., 2017). Additionally, to create an antagonistic environment through an increase in PH, Lactobacillus also competes for nutrients with said pathogens.

The exposure to commensal bacteria in the vagina seems to serve a protective purpose against pathogenic colonization. What if we're not exposed to vaginal fluid though? Children born by Cesarean seem to be more likely to develop diseases such as autism, obesity, asthma, allergies, and irritable bowel disease (Dunn, et. al., 2017). This may be due to two reasons. First, they're not being exposed to the commensal bacteria present in the vaginal fluids. Second, they're exposed to skin and oral microbes and any other organisms randomly present in the operating room (Dunn et. al., 2017). Being exposed to random microorganisms can lead to unpredictable consequences. This is particularly dangerous because they haven't been colonized by any commensal bacteria that can help ward off pathogens.

These facts are evidenced by the difference between the child's and mother's microbiomes. During the first six months after birth, an infant's microbiome should resemble their mother's. When a child is born by Cesarean, it doesn't. This is a risk factor mainly during the first six months though. Afterwards, a child's microbiome will begin to differ from the mother's anyway (Dunn et. al., 2017). However, as you may know, these first months after birth are critical periods for the child's body development, and any hindrance during these periods can have catastrophic and long-term effects.

The idea is that we should be exposed and colonized by a large number of diverse bacteria in order to have a healthy functioning microbiome and immune system. The ratio between the bacteria in each person's gut differs. Everybody's microbiome is different, which is why it's difficult to recommend a single type of product for the general public. Increasing one type of bacteria might be good for you, but not the next person.

Our microbial biodiversity can be hindered by different external and internal factors.

You can think of your different microbiomes as cities. You have microbiomes in your vagina, in your gut, your stomach, and many more regions. Within these populated cities, you will find neighborhoods or niches. The problem is that there are limited amounts of nutrients that come into these systems and some of the groups eat the same food. This is when competition arises.

Lactobacillus has gained its status as a benevolent bacteria because it eats some of the same foods pathogens eat. It competes for those nutrients, therefore starving the more opportunistic organisms. The other way Lactobacillus protects us is by raising the acidity levels in the environment, and we have discussed how H. Pylori in the stomach has the opposite effect, which is lowering our PH levels. It's thought that increasing the amount of Lactobacillus could possibly mitigate Pylori overgrowth (Sanhueza et. al., 2015).

The kind of nutrients we make available for our microbiota can tip the scale in favor of our commensal organisms. At the same time, it's known that pathogens, like the fungi Candida Albicans, love refined sugars. Research shows that the more Candida Albicans we have, the more we'll crave sugar, which can influence our food preferences (Singh et. al., 2017).

Pathogens thrive on certain carbohydrates mainly because they're difficult to break down or digest, allowing carbohydrates to reach our colon intact. Poor digestion, due to low PH levels or not enough enzyme production, can lead to small intestine bacterial overgrowth (SIBO). SIBO means that a lot of undigested food has been reaching the colon and feeding the wrong type of organisms. These opportunistic pathogens then start to crawl upwards into our small intestine from our colon. Once they're in our small intestine, they start to steal nutrients from our enterocytes. Basically, our body is forced to compete for nutrients with these organisms.

What we eat can tip the scale in our favor or not, but there have been more extreme methods used to change the composition of a person's microbiome. Fecal microbiota transplants (FMT) or bacteriotherapy is a method that has been growing in popularity for the treatment of C. Difficile infections. This would be a case of bacterial diarrhea, which can be much more harmful than the shorter-lived viral diarrheas we commonly get.

Recent studies have compared FMTs efficacy against placebos and even probiotics yielding positive results (Hui, etl al., 2019). This means that clinical researchers have been using colonoscopies to put fresh stool into people's guts, and it has been working. It seems like the stools don't have to be fresh all the time either. You can freeze them and introduce frozen stool capsules too. The meta-analysis provided this last year has documented how reliable and safe the practice can be when the stool donors are properly screened. These studies, however, don't speak so well about the oral ingestion of probiotics.

Synowiec et. al. (2018) ran another recent study on FMT. This experiment was done on mice due to ethical limitations; their results were quite interesting. The study consisted of categorizing behavioral patterns in mice. One group of mice were classified as timid mice, and the others were more adventurous and risk-taking mice. There were differences noticed in the compositions of each mice group's microbiome. After having noticed that, researchers hypothesized that a mouse's behavior might be influenced by the composition of their gut microbiome. To prove this hypothesis, the researchers took one group of mice's fecal matter and transplanted it into the other. The results were that the once timid mice became adventurous and vice-versa.

These results are promising, exciting and interesting, but we still need to reproduce these results many more times on different subjects. Mice aren't small humans after all, so we can't assume that these findings will apply to us. This must be tested on other species and reproduced many times over before we finally decide to run human trials. We're quite far from being able to manipulate a person's personality through stool.

Trust me, if more research begins to show up on how stool can alter your behaviors, there will be those who will profit from these findings. People will sell you stool to quit drugs, stool to become successful, and even stool from a genius so you can become smarter. People will sell it even without understanding the underlying mechanisms, as long as there is some poor desperate soul to be taken advantage of.

We're not sure if this only works on mice or if the experiments had some kind of confirmation bias. Even if the findings are reproducible, it still doesn't make it a safe procedure. We don't know why this is happening, we just know there's a correlation. We don't know what combination of microorganisms and their metabolites makes a mouse timid or adventurous.

Our microbiome is made up of the microbiota and their products, and some microbiota are more beneficial than others. How beneficial an organism is can also be determined by what foods we make available to it. Some commensal bacteria may turn pathogenic if they're starved and forced to eat something other than what they usually consume. Once transformed, these microbes are called pathobionts.

We are colonized by benevolent bacteria in our mother's womb at birth, which helps us resist pathogenic colonization early on. Pathogens can thrive when we consume too much of a food that we're unable to digest easily; this is what is meant by the term food intolerance. Continuous consumption of foods you're intolerant to can lead to SIBO and general colon dysbiosis.

You should now have a general understanding of how the microbiome is constituted. Next, we're going to explore the specific interactions it may have with several diseases.

CHAPTER 03
BLOATING AND DIGESTION

We're going to begin to talk about some of the abnormalities that can arise from having an unhealthy lifestyle and, therefore, an unhealthy microbiome. Some of the main indicators of an unhealthy microbiome are a lack of microbial biodiversity and low levels of short-chain fatty acid (SCFA) production.

The gut-associated lymphoid tissue (GALT) is one of the largest immune organs in our body. This is the mucus layer of cells on your intestinal wall where your villi are. Its job is to determine what we should let into our bloodstream or not. It keeps out microorganisms and undigested food molecules. This is the immune system we will be referring to in this chapter.

Bloating & Inflammation

To better understand the microbiome's impact on our body, we should explore another one of the microbiome's proposed functions. The microbiota within our gut is thought to share a symbiotic relationship with us, meaning that we help each other survive and adapt to our environment. Our microbiome teaches our immune system not to overreact when it comes across microorganisms by exposing it to small harmless quantities of the microbes. Our microbiome helps our immune system build a certain tolerance to pathogens, food molecules, and waste products so that we're not overly sensitive to them. Having a fragile or sensitive immune system is what leads to allergies (Belkaid & Hand, 2014).

The introduction of commensal bacteria through a mother's breast milk accustoms a child's immune system to the commensal bacteria and their metabolites. This makes it so our system does not try to attack our commensal bacteria, and it helps calibrate our immune system to react appropriately to food molecules. Our immune system's response causes inflammation to isolate the intruder and keep them from coming in contact with any more of our tissue.

This may explain the reason why there's a correlation between being born by C-section and developing food allergies. Our immune system might not have been stimulated enough by microbes, which can make our immune system overly sensitive, causing chronic inflammation. The issue with chronic inflammation is that it only leads to more inflammation and other complications. No matter what the reason for inflammation is, whether it be genetic, due to an unhealthy lifestyle, or dysbiosis (could be all three), it can lead to further complications if not addressed.

Chronic inflammation can loosen the tight junctures between the cells in your intestinal lining or lumen. If the junctures aren't tight enough, undigested food molecules and even microorganisms can get through into your bloodstream, causing more immune responses and more inflammation.

This condition is called leaky gut. It means that the mucosal wall of your intestine is too permeable and not selective enough; it's unable to do its job at filtering what comes into your bloodstream. Once in your bloodstream, these microorganisms or undigested molecules can be transported anywhere else in your body. This is why theories have risen around the more mysterious autoimmune diseases of our era, like arthritis and fibromyalgia. The idea is that if you have suffered from chronic inflammation in your gut for years, harmful unfiltered materials could be transported to your hand's joints, for example, which would be an example of the autoimmune response described by people suffering from arthritis. There's still much research to be done on these correlations between leaky gut syndrome and our autoimmune diseases, and at first glance it does make sense.

Gas and bloating are ways your body is trying to communicate to you that something is going wrong. Gas should only be looked at as a sign of an issue if you feel it has become excessive. Gas is produced mainly in our colon, and this occurs due to bacterial fermentation. Undigested foods make it to our colon where our microbiota processes them; then the metabolites released are what makes us gassy.

There are some indigestible foods that we consume which cause bloating. Why would we put something in our body that it can't process? Isn't that the definition of the word poison? A poison is something our body can't metabolize in an appropriate time period, or when it does metabolize, it is turned into harmful toxins. One example of these characteristics is alcohol. Alcohol is used to sterilize equipment, so naturally, it kills bacteria indiscriminately. Still, it feeds pathogenic fungi that seek it, such as Candida Albicans, and of course, it isn't metabolized efficiently by our liver.

So if you're experiencing gas or bloating, then it's most likely because your body is not able to process a specific type of food you're ingesting. The best way to find out what it is by removing a few of the things you think could be affecting you, and then start adding them back into your life one by one to see which one has that bloating reaction on you.

Otherwise, continuing to eat foods that your body is unable to metabolize efficiently can lead to irritable bowel disease, obesity, or even food allergies. For the time being, we don't fully understand what causes irritable bowel disease, but what we can do is change the way we're eating.

Whether you're not able to process foods for genetic or microbial reasons, in the end, you're still causing inflammation, and that's something that needs to be addressed immediately.

Another reason you may be experiencing gas and bloating is due to malabsorption. The majority of malabsorption cases occur either due to poor digestion in the stomach, lack of mucosal cells in the gut, or a loss in our capacity to move the nutrients throughout our bloodstream. Malabsorption leads to malnourishment. You can be malnourished and still be overweight because it just means you're not extracting the nutrients essential for your bodily functions. For example, if your pancreas is not getting the nutrients it needs to produce the enzymatic cells required to digest and absorb nutrients, you will end up with an even greater case of malabsorption. It's a self-fulfilling cycle.

If you're not absorbing the nutrient into your intestinal wall, something will. This is why malabsorption can lead to gas and bloating. When you don't absorb your nutrients, the bacteria in your gut colon will, and the products they produce will cause you to bloat.

Some of the ways that malabsorption occurs is through prolonged use of antibiotics, surgery, or irritable bowel disease. Irritable bowel disease (IBD) is an umbrella term that includes any sort of chronic inflammation in your gut. A change in our diet in the last few decades may provide some clues as to why these diseases have emerged. IBS is underdiagnosed since many people fail to recognize the symptoms, and because of its chronic nature. It isn't something you would typically go to the hospital for. Even though it's underdiagnosed, we're still aware that it affects at least 11% of the global population (Canavan & Card, 2014).

There are disproportionately high correlations between people with IBS and other autoimmune diseases, such as fibromyalgia, arthritis, chronic fatigue, and even psychiatric disorders. About 50% of people who report IBS also report one of the previously mentioned conditions (Canavan & Card, 2014).

IBS, along with these other autoimmune diseases, is poorly understood by the scientific community. Some researchers even go as far as to call them "functional somatic symptoms." This conveys the notion that the illnesses are highly psychological in nature and symptoms we're expressing throughout our body don't truly have a physiological root, but a psychological one. The theory is that these symptoms are born out of the way we deal with stress. This just adds another layer of complexity into the issue of gut health.

Serotonin and dopamine play large roles in our mood regulation. Most serotonin and a large part of our body's dopamine is produced in our gut. These endorphins are the chemicals your brain releases when you look at a sunset, when you pet your dog, when you make love to your partner and when you eat delicious food. They're nature's feel-good chemicals. Dopamine is nature's way of telling you, you're on the right path. An example of this is found in deer. Deer can sniff out water a long distance away, and when they catch the scent of water, their brain releases dopamine. This gets them excited and motivates them to continue searching. This is adaptive and very useful for any living organism's survival. In the same sense, when you feel you're on the right path like you're following your calling or purpose in life, dopamine will also be released.

These chemicals are fundamental to our sense of wellbeing and fulfillment. There is a gut-brain connection; in fact, the gut is called the "second brain" by many. This is because the enteric nervous system is directly connected to our central nervous system through the vagus nerve. In some sense, our gut has its own brain, and a lot of its functions are independent from our brain. If the connection between your mind and your gut were to be severed, you would still pass bowel movements and perform other intestinal functions.

These facts allow us to imagine why depression and anxiety disorders are present in more than half the people who report inflammatory issues in their gut. It's clear that conditions like depression and anxiety coexist with IBD, but we don't know which one comes first; it's much like the chicken and the egg dilemma. Neurotic disorders worsen IBD, and IBD can worsen your depression and anxiety.

One of the mechanisms by which depression and anxiety influences our gut health is through an excessive secretion of cortisol (the stress hormone). The microbes in our gut have evolved to detect changes in our bodies and respond to them. They respond to the chronic increases in our cortisol levels, and specific pathogens seem to thrive in cortisol rich environments (Foster, Rynaman, & Cryan, 2017).

Stress tips the scale in favor of pathogens that compete for nutrients with Lactobacillus Plantarum. This strain of Lactobacillus seems to be correlated with increased levels of serotonin and dopamine, which provides us with a clue to what occurs in this type of dysbiosis. Less serotonin and dopamine are transported and synthesized (Foster, Rynaman, & Cryan, 2017) and, since the pathogens thrive on cortisol, they may even stimulate the increased production of cortisol. Again, this is a cycle because stress will lead to more cortisol production. In return, inflammation will happen as our immune system tries to fight off the pathogens and their toxic metabolites. Like I said, local inflammation in your gut may cause loose junctions or a leaky gut, which will allow more toxins and microorganisms in, firing even more autoimmune responses.

Chronic activation of our immune system from chronic inflammation puts the body into a state of constant fatigue. Your body is expending energy trying to keep out the toxic molecules that are coming in, making you feel tired. Being tired makes you irritable and less motivated and also anxious, stressed, or depressed.

This gut-brain connection we're learning more and more about gives a whole new meaning to old expressions like "I have a gut feeling." It seems like people were truly onto something with that expression. Again, it's hard to tell which came first, but it's clear these conditions coexist, and they reinforce each other.

Emulsifiers & IBD

Emulsifiers are food additives found in processed foods. They're used to bind lipids with water and create a consistent and pleasurable texture. Some examples of foods that use this can be mayonnaise, chocolate syrup, many creamy sauces, and dressings.

This is going to be one of the main reasons we should avoid processed foods. Emulsifiers are detergents, meaning that they bind with oils/lipids. Our intestinal wall is made out of mucosa, and this mucus has oils in it. When the emulsifiers interact with our intestinal walls, they allow microbiota to insert themselves in them. When this happens, our body releases an immune response that creates antimicrobial chemicals (Chassaing et. al., 2017). If our body continuously has this immune response, not only would we be suffering from chronic inflammation, but we would also be reducing our microbial biodiversity through the excessive release of antimicrobial chemicals. This means that inflammation directly reduces our microbiome's diversity, which in turn, will only lead to more inflammation.

Our body tries to fight off the intruders the emulsifiers let in through the deterioration of our intestinal wall. The way we stop more organisms from getting in is by creating inflammation, which will tightly seal any gateways into our body (Chassaing et. al., 2017). We rather have inflammation than allow gut fungi to colonize one of our other organs, and they do reach our other organs, the result can potentially be fatal. Finally, in our attempt to kill off the bacteria that are intruding, we release antimicrobial chemicals that, when released excessively, kill off our good bacteria as well.

When making your purchases at the grocery store, you want to look at the labels and stop buying two main emulsifiers: carboxymethylcellulose (CMC) and polysorbate 80. Perhaps it would be good to do more research as time goes on because companies can get tricky with their labeling and even slightly change compounds in the emulsifiers just to be able to change the name. This is also why it's hard to spot high fructose corn syrup (HFCS) on labels these days. Emulsifiers can lead to chronic inflammation, but even if they're not the cause, they will only exacerbate your symptoms.

Warning Signs

There are a few factors that you should take into consideration if you want to know whether you're at risk of developing IBS or not. Chronic inflammation leads to disease, so we must pay attention to any signs of possible inflammation. You want to be paying attention to any sensation of discomfort you may feel after eating or defecating.

After eating, some common signs of inflammation can be bloating, excessive gas, cramps, and an overwhelming urgency to go to the bathroom. All these can be looked at as signs that something you're eating is not being metabolized by your body adequately. Bloating can be seen as a feeling of being full and heavy, while cramping is described as a sensation of tightness and constriction.

After defecating, you may also feel bloating and cramping. Tenesmus is another sensation indicative of possible inflammation. This sensation is described as a feeling of incomplete evacuation, where you feel like you weren't able to get it all out, but you're unable to continue evacuating. Discomfort after eating and during or after defecating is noteworthy. This is the first set of criteria we'll use as signs of inflammation.

The second factor you want to bring to awareness is stool frequency. You want to be defecating at least three times per week, but no more than three times per day.

Finally, stool consistency and changes in your stools will be signs of possible faulty digestion and malabsorption.

This is the most commonly used chart to this day. On one end, you will find the stool that reflects constipation, and on the other side, you have diarrhea.

Bristol Stool Chart

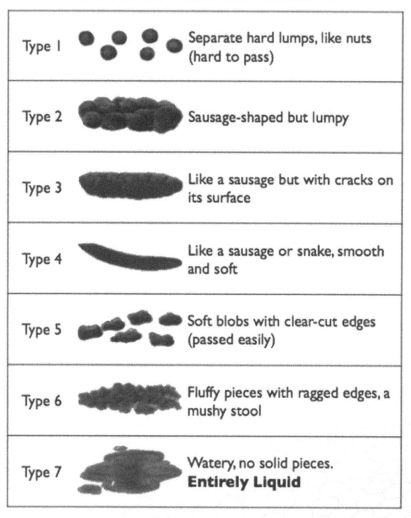

Type 1	Separate hard lumps, like nuts (hard to pass)
Type 2	Sausage-shaped but lumpy
Type 3	Like a sausage but with cracks on its surface
Type 4	Like a sausage or snake, smooth and soft
Type 5	Soft blobs with clear-cut edges (passed easily)
Type 6	Fluffy pieces with ragged edges, a mushy stool
Type 7	Watery, no solid pieces. **Entirely Liquid**

Figure 2: Bristol Stool Chart

We will be using this chart to discuss changes in stool consistency that you may experience. The best way to go about this process is to keep track of your stools; perhaps you can download an app that can help you, or you can simply write it down on your cellphone or journal.

When you register one of your stools, you want to write down the time, date, and stool type. This is what will be required for you to find out if there's really an issue. You have to do this for at least three months. You can also record the sensations that came afterwards as well. If you want to take it a step further, you can write down what you eat on a daily basis and try to correlate it to the sensations and stool types experienced.

You want to be around stool types 3 and 4 with no sensation of tenesmus. That's the description of healthy bowel movements. For changes in stool consistency, you want less than 25% of your stools to be above type 4 and less than 25% of them to be below type 3.

Now, after the three month period, you will come to know if there's a problem. If you experienced discomfort, changes in stool frequency, changes in stool consistency, or tenesmus at least once per week for three months, then you can start to believe there's an issue. If you do spot an issue, then you should probably adhere to the following guidelines, or perhaps even if you don't have a problem, these recommendations can become preventive measures.

You should most definitely increase your fiber intake to 30 grams per day. We're talking about leafy greens and some grains such as lentils. This is mainly because we don't metabolize fiber; it's food for our colon's good bacteria. If the organisms in our colon don't have food, they can either begin to cannibalize the mucus of our intestinal wall, since it's made up of sugars, or they can even start to wander up into our small intestine to compete with our absorptive cells for nutrients.

We will discuss the mechanisms by which fiber is key to a healthy lifestyle in the following chapter. Lactose and coffee may not be the causes behind your inflammation, but once you do have chronic inflammation, they can act as irritants. Your body may have become sensitive to these foods with the deterioration of your intestinal lining. Cutting these out at least for a while will help you recover, and eventually adding them into your diet later to see how your body reacts may be necessary.

One final recommendation would be a diet low in fermentable oligosaccharides, disaccharides, monosaccharides, and polyols (FODMAP). These are short-chain carbohydrates that are poorly metabolized by people. They're fermented in our colon by our microbiota, but the byproducts produced causes inflammation, bloating, and gas (Zanetti, Rogero, & Atzinegen, 2018).

Some of these foods' characteristics include poor absorption of nutrients since we lack sufficient enzymes to break down these molecules, and being too large to be transported into the bloodstream as a whole.

These foods have high osmotic activity, meaning that they move water into our intestines exacerbating the existing symptoms we experience with IBS.

Each person can have different resistances or sensitivities to the foods in this category, so the first approach would be to eliminate them all for about a month and then begin to monitor your body as you introduce one food type at a time. Reintroduce each food type for three days in smaller proportions to see how you feel. If you feel fine, then increase it to the normal portion of the specific food you would usually have.

Here are the food types that are included on the list. You may notice that some of them are rich in fiber, yet the issue is how fermentable these items are.

I'm not saying these should all be avoided, but it is known that some people can be sensitive to some of these, leading them to chronic inflammation. This is why each person has to discover what is affecting them. All our microbiomes are different.

High FODMAP Foods

Vegetables & Legumes

- Onion
- Garlic
- Asparagus
- Cauliflower
- Cabbage
- Mushrooms
- Beans

Fruit

- Ripe Bananas
- Apples
- Mangos
- Avocados

Meat

- Processed meat (i.e. sausages)

Dairy

- Cow's milk
- Soy milk
- Sheep's milk
- Goat's milk
- Icecream
- Sour cream
- Cream cheese

Sugar

- High fructose corn syrup (HFCS)

In order to begin to identify some of the foods that may be causing us inflammation, we must be aware of the composition of our industrialized processed foods. Reading labels must become a regular practice for you.

One of the issues with restrictive diet plans like this one is that they can reduce your microbial diversity. This is why you only want to remove these foods temporarily if you have already spotted that you're having chronic bowel irritation. This diet is only a means to identify the causes of your inflammation.

Cortisol & IBD

Cortisol is one of the main hormones associated with the way our body reacts to stress. Cortisol production is stimulated through the activation of a particular part of our autonomic nervous system. As the name implies, our autonomic nervous system takes care of most of our body's automatic processes like digestion.

The part of our autonomic nervous system that is activated during a stress response is called the sympathetic nervous system. Our sympathetic nervous system is responsible for feelings of arousal, alert states of mind, and stress responses. Evolutionarily, we should be grateful to our sympathetic system since it's responsible for the fight or flight state described in survival situations. We need energy and focus to be able to fight a predator or run away. This is why adrenaline and cortisol are released in moments of stress. The chemicals previously mentioned are released whether the stress we perceive is real or imaginary.

In our modern era, we're not in survival situations as often as we used to be. The stress we experience nowadays is chronic rather than acute. Many people spend a large part of their day feeling financial pressures and worrying about meeting deadlines. On top of that, you can add emotional disturbances to these ubiquitous stress factors, and we end up with excessively high levels of cortisol.

Whenever you're stressed, you are activating your sympathetic nervous system, which in turn deactivates your parasympathetic nervous system. Sympathetic nervous system activation increases your LDL cholesterol levels, blood pressure, and cortisol blood levels.

On the other hand, your parasympathetic nervous system is involved in regenerative processes, meaning the creation of new cells. This nervous system is responsible for healing and reconstruction.

We're going to be talking about how cortisol is tied to obesity, mental health, and sleep in subsequent chapters. In each chapter, I'm going to give you an activity that can help you activate your parasympathetic nervous system or at least reduce your cortisol levels.

Prolonged activation of the sympathetic nervous system leads to overall higher concentrations of cortisol in our body, which then stimulates your immune system to produce inflammatory cytokines. These cytokines are one of the main factors involved in the pathogenesis (birth of disease) of IBD (Mawdsley & Rampton, 2016). Beneficial bacteria in our colon produce SCFAs such as butyrate and acetate, which can suppress the productions of cytokines.

The goal here is to reduce the amount of cortisol our body produces. One way to do this is by lowering our brain's reactivity to stress. A person's reactivity to stress is tied to a person's resilience, or their ability to adapt to changing environments. Let's say you got broken up with, got into a car crash, or lost your job. All these changes in your environment will elicit a stress response from you. Your sympathetic nervous system will activate since you need to be alert and ready to look for a new job, for example. The issue lies in being alert all the time, being overly stressed without the ability to relax.

Some people have a real hard time turning off their responses to stress. They may stay angry or depressed about something longer than other people. This inability to let go maybe because cortisol levels linger in their bodies for longer, even after the stressing event has passed. This is what is meant by "reactivity to stress"; it is how long our body keeps cortisol levels increased.

Physical exercise seems to be correlated with our reactivity to stress (Mawdsley & Rampton, 2016) and allows us to adjust to the curveballs life throws at us with ease. If our cortisol levels stabilize quickly after a stressful situation, it means that our body will, in general, exhibit lower cortisol levels throughout the day.

Along with the fact that exercise helps us reduce cortisol, it also stimulates our body's dopamine secretion. Whenever you endure a painful experience, your body will try to compensate for the pain you feel with dopamine. It's your body's attempt to alleviate pain. It's like your very own natural pain killer. Similarly, when you eat something really spicy, you may get a headrush, and that's because of the dopamine that's being released due to the intense pain felt. Through the pain of exercising your muscles, working out will release dopamine, which will in turn activate your parasympathetic nervous system, stimulating the secretion of somatotropin. Somatotropin is referred to as the human growth hormone (HGH), which is why our parasympathetic nervous system is involved in healing and regeneration.

There are two options when it comes to exercise. You can either do a milder cardiovascular exercise for about 20 minutes (i.e., jogging or riding a bike), or you can do high-intensity short interval exercise. The second option may not be for everyone, but if you can do it, you should. It consists of high-intensity exercises for intervals of 30 seconds or less. This can be sprinting for 15 seconds at maximum speed or doing 10 repetitions with your maximum weight limit. You want to carry out short intervals of intense exercise.

Putting ourselves in stressful or painful situations, which is what happens when we exercise, increases our tolerance to discomfort and stress. This means our body may produce less cortisol since our threshold to pain will be increased.

You must pay attention to the warning signs your body gives you, whether it be bloating, gas, or diarrhea. By now, you should realize that diarrhea doesn't have to be extreme. You don't have to be "peeing out of your bottom side" all day, to the point that you can't walk for diarrhea to be considered a warning sign.

Inflammation can lead to disease and is usually caused by either eating foods our body is sensitive to or excessive amounts of stress. Finding what these foods are is essential to prevent ourselves from having IBD. Remember, IBD coexists with depression, obesity, and sleep disorders, so we're not just talking about avoiding gas and diarrhea here. Finally, exercise will be a mechanism by which you can lower the amount of cortisol in your body, which is also essential to mitigating the symptoms experienced in IBD.

In the following chapter, we will look at two more ways to combat inflammatory and metabolic diseases.

CHAPTER 04
PROBIOTICS AND FIBER

Dietary fiber and probiotics are two of the most potent tools we have at our disposal. Pathogens and commensal bacteria in normal conditions live in a state of dynamic equilibrium within our gut, and we must do everything we can to keep it this way. In this chapter, we'll see what recent scientific discoveries have to say about these potent tools.

Probiotics

Probiotics are sets of live microorganisms cultured specifically for humans; these microorganisms have grown quite popular recently. You may ingest probiotics through freeze-dried supplemental capsules or through foods that have been fermented by microorganisms. One of the most potent foods containing probiotics is thought to be yogurt. By ingesting probiotics, we're allowing either new bacteria to colonize us or reinforcing the communities that already reside within our gut. Our commensal bacteria are thought to act as a bacterial barrier, and they're one of our first lines of defense against the external world. If you think about it, our gastrointestinal tract is the biggest organ that interfaces with the external world along with our skin. Therefore, barricading the entrances to our bodies with bacterial walls might not be such a bad idea.

The methods by which we expose our body to probiotics are in question though. It's still up to debate what the best method might be. Is it best to consume freeze-dried supplements, get the bacteria naturally from our diet, or perhaps eat some mud, as many children do? Just kidding on that last part. Which species should we be ingesting more of? How much of it? These are all valid questions that we should be asking ourselves before we go out and make a purchase.

First, let's debunk the yogurt industry's messages. Most yogurt contains probiotics; this much is true. How many active or live probiotics survive the processing is a whole other question. Let's say that all the probiotics survive, though. Even if that's the case, the amount of probiotics present in yogurt is still quite inconsequential. You would have to ingest large quantities of yogurt before you could meet the number of probiotics you receive from a supplement. Also, most yogurts are high in emulsifiers and/or refined sugars.

Emulsifiers reduce the amount of bacteria that survive in the mixture. Refined sugars can help feed your pathogenic bacteria which compete with the probiotics you want to colonize you. So, in the end, you are consuming more probiotics for the pathogens, which completely defeats the purpose of consuming probiotics in the first place.

Prebiotics are foods that help feed certain sets of microorganisms.

So if yogurt isn't the answer, we should all consume probiotics through supplements. Well, there isn't any evidence for significant risk factors in consuming probiotic supplements. So if you can afford them, then take them!

There is one primary concern when it comes to the supplement industry, which is that most probiotics are marketed as dietary supplements. Since they're not sold as drugs that can treat any specific illnesses, they don't need the FDA's approval. Dietary supplements may not be able to say they cure a disease, but they can talk about how they affect your body. These statements don't have to be scientifically validated, which is why we must be responsible and inform ourselves before making our purchases.

Let's remember that probiotics are living organisms. These organisms are usually rendered dormant in their capsules through a process of freeze-drying. The way they're stored, packaged, and shipped is crucial to their survival. Taking dead microbes wouldn't really help your gut become more biodiverse. Moisture and heat are to be avoided at all times, as either of these factors could awaken the dormant microbes only to have them die from a lack of nutrients.

The most popular types of bacteria that have been deemed as generally regarded as safe (GRAS) are the Bifidobacterium and Lactobacillus genera. The strains under these genera are considered optimal since they're acid-resistant, which allows them to reach the gut by surviving your stomach acids. They're also able to adhere to our intestinal wall easily where they may colonize us. Once they've colonized us, the metabolites produced by them may create a hostile environment where pathogens such as Salmonella and C. Difficile aren't able to thrive (Thantsha & Mbiriri, 2012).

Probiotics act as a bacterial wall by sticking to the intestinal lining. The fact that they grow there keeps other pathogens from colonizing us. This is evident in individuals who, for some reason, have had to take excessive amounts of antibiotics, flushing their intestinal flora clean. Antibiotics don't discriminate the good from the harmful bacteria, so when the good bacteria is diminished, it leaves us exposed to C. Difficile infections, for example.

C. Difficile is a pathogen that is known for its ability to produce destructive bacterial diarrhea. Bacterial diarrhea is different from viral diarrhea. Infectious diarrhea can be a more gradual process and, depending on your gut's health, may not be cured on its own. Symptoms range from blood in your stools to diarrhea, which occurs three to ten times a day. The main difference between viral and bacterial diarrhea is that viral diarrhea doesn't cause inflammation that destroys your intestinal lining. In contrast, bacterial infections do destroy your lining, which is why blood is present.

Infectious diarrhea can be life-threatening, particularly in the elderly. Coincidentally, a person's intestinal biodiversity begins to diminish as they get older; this may be one reason why they're more susceptible to the infection. Administering Bifidobacterium genera through antibiotics has proven to reverse these infections in many cases (Thantsha & Mbiriri, 2012).

An alternative to taking freeze-dried probiotics through supplements is to include probiotic-rich foods in your diet. Fermented fruits and vegetables can provide a diverse and large quantity of microorganisms. Kimchi, sauerkraut, kombucha, and chutney are some of the most popular foods that are recommended. Just like with yogurt, you want to watch the amount of sugar you're ingesting. There are quite a few mainstream kombucha products with extremely high sugar levels.

Whether you decide to get your probiotics from supplements or through a diverse diet is up to you. That's all based on your lifestyle and whether you have the time to procure or make fermented foods. It doesn't hurt to do both, since the evidence shows that we need as much diversity in our gut as we can get. It's not so much about increasing a single strain, but having as many as you can. As for how necessary taking a supplement might be, that's still up to debate.

Dietary Fiber

We previously mentioned the term prebiotics. This is mainly what fiber is; it's food for your good bacteria. Prebiotics are substances that feed commensal bacteria and are metabolized into beneficial or harmless byproducts. Dietary fiber is made of plant cells and can't be produced by our body, so we have to acquire it through our diet.

Fiber isn't digested by the cells in our body. Instead, it goes straight to our colon to be digested by our commensal bacteria. The byproducts born from this are the SCFAs, as we mentioned. If we don't have a lot of fiber in our diet, our commensal bacteria will be forced to adapt and look for alternative food sources.

Most fast food items need to have their fiber removed in order to improve their shelf-life. At the same time, these foods are also high in refined sugars. Junk foods make it so our commensal bacteria end up having to switch to sugar as a food source. This turns our commensal bacteria into pathobionts; pathobionts are bacteria that were once commensal and became pathogenic due to changes in their environment. These pathobionts eat the sugar since there's not enough fiber for them, and then they turn the sugar into inflammation-causing metabolites (Rinezi et. al., 2020).

This is why the idea of benevolent bacteria isn't 100% accurate. Our microbiotas' role really depends on our lifestyle and what kinds of other microbes we are exposed to and colonized by. This may be the reason why we see cases in which probiotics don't really do much for some people.

The consensus for microbial equilibrium is less than 25 grams of sugar per day. Most people in the United States are consuming about 80-100 grams of sugar per day (Rienzi et. al., 2020). Eating at least 30 grams of fiber will ensure that our commensal bacteria won't switch food sources.

Fiber-Rich Options:
- Lentils
- Leafy Greens
- Apples
- Avocados
- Quinoa
- Artichokes
- Sweet potatoes
- Dark chocolate

One last comment on fiber is that fiber stimulates leptin release, which is the hormone responsible for satiety. This is why eating fiber-rich foods can make you feel satisfied for longer. Processed sugars, on the other hand, don't stimulate the release of this hormone. This may be why we say, "there's always room for dessert." Overeating isn't easy. You'll feel sick and want to vomit if you try to overeat fiber-rich foods, mainly because leptin is able to do its job.

In the following chapter, we will look into what is known about the mechanism that leads to obesity and how our microbiome may influence those mechanisms. Sugar, processed foods, and stress will continue to be key points to focus on through our journey of understanding and healing.

CHAPTER 05
FAT LOSS AND OBESITY

Obesity has risen to epidemic proportions in our era, and coincidentally, this story links back to our tale about microbes and hygiene.

As we improved our standards of hygiene, so did our life expectancy (Fung, 2016). We began to live into our later years, mainly because we weren't dying from bacterial infections anymore; tuberculosis became a thing of the past. An increase in life expectancy allowed us to live long enough for us to develop coronary heart disease. Coronary heart disease became one of our primary concerns. We were under the impression that a heart disease epidemic had started (Fung, 2016). So our attention shifted over to dietary fat. This was when you started seeing all those trendy low-fat products arise. Fat became public enemy number one.

If we're not going to consume our calories from fat, then where would we get them? Protein? There aren't that many options since there are only three main macronutrients; protein, carbohydrates, and lipids (fats).

Protein could not be the answer since high protein products like dairy and meat also contain high amounts of fat, so the solution was carbohydrates. Sugar and all sorts of refined grains became our main alternative to fat. This, of course, happened because we thought that all fat was bad and would lead to heart disease. Sugar was also put into these fat-free products to make them taste better because low-fat food didn't taste good at all. At one point in our history, it was thought that processed food was an improved version of real food. This idea came to be because refined sugars and grains were low on fats; therefore, they must be good since they're not fattening.

Fat was demonized in 1977 by the U.S. government, and the decision that fat

The Secrets To Improve Bloating, Digestion, Anxiety And Fat Loss

was causing obesity was not made by the scientific community but by government decree (Fung, 2016). People were asked to remove their fat intake, and they did, which is why we're in the situation we're in today. Fat consumption was reduced from 40% to 30%, while carbohydrate consumption was increased to make up 60% of the calories we consume on a daily basis.

Food and drink companies have grown dramatically since the 1970s, from mid-size companies to multinational powerhouses (Gardner, 2020). These companies now fund a large part of nutritional research, in the United States at least, pushing their agenda and applying a lot of the same tactics the tobacco and pharmaceutical industries have in the past. Tactics such as biased scientific research are used to influence public opinion.

The idea that the food and drink industry doesn't have our general wellbeing at heart sounds like a conspiracy theory. You could argue that there are so many products to choose from nowadays that they couldn't all be from less than reputable sources. The issue is that 90% of the food distribution and marketing is controlled by only 10 companies in the United States: Kraft, Coca-Cola, Nestle, Kelloggs, Pepsico, Johnson & Johnson, P&G, Unilever, MARS, and General Mills. This means that the policies behind the products we're consuming aren't really that diverse (Gardner, 2020).

It was thought that fast food would help liberate us from having to cook, so we could spend more time doing other activities in life. This was the birth of fast food, and in this regard, it has been successful. People do spend a lot less time cooking and eating.

Processed food can be looked at as fiberless food with long shelf lives. Shelf lives are extended by emulsifiers, additives, salt, and by removing fiber from the products. One final ingredient is prevalent in our processed foods to mask all the sour, bitter, and salty tastes: sugar.

Sugar exists in nature as a way to tell our body that the item we're ingesting is safe to eat. There aren't any sweet foods in nature that are severely poisonous. Therefore, it was adaptive for us to develop an attraction towards sweet tastes.

The fact the food and drink industries have increasingly added larger amounts of sugar into our food isn't accidental; they know what they're doing and why. Sugar is just as addictive as alcohol or tobacco, and it lures our dopamine reward systems in the same way. All the signs we look for in other drug addictions are also present in sugar consumption. Craving, tolerance, and withdrawal are the three factors by which we determine addiction to a substance. Paul Van der Velpen (as cited in WN, 2014) claims that sugar is one of the most dangerous drugs of our time. Paul is Amsterdam's public health chief, so he would know a thing or two about dangerous drugs.

Our brain is wired to release dopamine when we eat. Have you ever tried eating the same meal for a prolonged period of time? Let's say you have fish and salad every day; eventually, the dopamine your brain releases towards the meal reduces because our brain has trained you to want to seek out new meals. This is a mechanism that stimulates us to keep a balanced and diverse diet. Every time we switch things up and eat something different, our brain releases increased levels of dopamine, making us enjoy the novel tastes a bit more. In other words, this is why we get tired of eating the same foods all the time.

The issue with sugar is that our brain's dopamine release doesn't decrease over time; we don't get tired of it, in other words. We do grow tolerant of it and are able to consume larger amounts of sugar without getting sick of it. The fact that dopamine continues to be released even after continuous ingestion of sugar is what makes it so addictive. The addictive side of processed foods is mainly due to the added sugar these foods contain. This is great for our consumerist economic system because it needs us to keep consuming.

Activating the pleasure centers in our brain is one way that food companies get us to buy more; another way is by making us feel satiated for shorter periods of time. This is because fiberless products release a lot less leptin, as discussed.

It's thought that the obesity epidemic occurred due to our gluttonous disposition and that, as a society, we've become more self-indulging and lazy. People may tell us that we've been on a constant moral descent. The truth is, we have increased the amount of calories we ingest in general, but the increase has not been significant, and by no means is it proportional to how obese we've become.

We've been programmed by the idea that we gain weight because we consume more calories than we spend (Fung, 2016). The mantra up until now has been "eat less, move more." The idea that eating less and moving more is all it takes to combat obesity makes it sound like we've all become overindulging and lazy. This idea turned obesity into a moral failing when, in fact, 70% of what makes people obese comes from nature/genetics as opposed to nurture/lifestyle. Science isn't saying that you're destined to be obese. You can change that. It's only saying that there are people who are more likely to be obese.

Fung references a study by Dr. Stunkard (2006 as cited by Fung, 2016) where adoptive children whose genome had been studied were introduced into adoptive families with varying lifestyles and eating habits. This study showed that the adoptive family's lifestyle had little to no impact on the children's weight. In the study, it was noticed that some of the fattest adoptees had the thinnest adoptive families. Genetics may explain obesity in household environments, but it doesn't explain why a whole society is becoming increasingly obese (Fung, 2016).

Fung (2016), in his enlightening work on obesity, asks us to think about why there are obese physicians. Why would your doctor be obese? Most people associate obesity with a lack of discipline but if you think about it, going to medical school takes an enormous amount of discipline, so that can't be the sole reason. What is being proposed is that the approach and knowledge we have about obesity is incomplete.

Obesity is a hormonal imbalance, not a moral failing; it's not something that can be overcome simply by eating less or moving to a restrictive diet.

Insulin: Energy Storage Hormone

Dietary guidelines have been asking us to control our calorie intake as a way to stay healthy. This mandate shifts our attention from the real issue. It makes us believe that a calorie is a calorie. If a calorie were a calorie, then you could get your 2000 calories per day from cheesecake and soft drinks or from salad and fish, and gain the same amount of weight. This would make sense since you're consuming the same amount of calories. The problem is that different calories are metabolized differently by our body, so a calorie is not just a calorie (Fung, 2016).

The message here isn't that all carbohydrates are bad, as this has been disproven. Some carbs have a different insulin response than others; you can consult different glycemic indexes to get a good idea of which foods spike your insulin levels the most (See Fig. 3)

Glycemic Index

Low GI (<55), Medium GI (56-69) and High GI (70>)

Grains / Starchs		Vegetables		Fruits		Dairy		Proteins	
Rice Bran	27	Asparagus	15	Grapefruit	25	Low-Fat Yogurt	14	Peanuts	21
Bran Cereal	42	Broccoli	15	Apple	38	Plain Yogurt	14	Beans, Dried	40
Spaghetti	42	Celery	15	Peach	42	Whole Milk	27	Lentils	41
Corn, sweet	54	Cucumber	15	Orange	44	Soy Milk	30	Kidney Beans	41
Wild Rice	57	Lettuce	15	Grape	46	Fat-Free Milk	32	Split Peas	45
Sweet Potatoes	61	Peppers	15	Banana	54	Skim Milk	32	Lima Beans	46
White Rice	64	Spinach	15	Mango	56	Chocolate Milk	35	Chickpeas	47
Cous Cous	65	Tomatoes	15	Pineapple	66	Fruit Yogurt	36	Pinto Beans	55
Whole Wheat	71	Chickpeas	33	Watermelon	72	Ice Cream	61	Black-Eyed Beans	59
Bread		Cooked Carrots	39						
Muesli	80								
Baked Potatoes	85								
Oatmeal	87								
Taco Shells	97								
White Bread	100								
Bagel, White	103								

Figure 3: Glycemic Index

Calories are the last thing you need to look at on a nutritional label. The idea that a calorie is a calorie makes us believe those excess calories are the culprits behind obesity and not what we eat and when we eat it.

Different calories are associated with different insulin responses. Insulin levels are correlated with weight gain. If your blood insulin levels are always high, you will gain weight (Fung, 2016). You will gain weight no matter what you eat or how much you exercise as long as your insulin levels are high. The weight you gain from high insulin levels is mainly around your waist and near your organs since it's visceral fat.

Insulin is secreted in our pancreas as a response to increased glucose (blood sugar) levels. Our glucose levels spike when we eat, so insulin's role is to signal our body to store the energy we're receiving in our muscles, bones, adipose tissue, and liver. The mechanisms by which insulin makes us fat are quite complex and not fully understood yet, but the correlations are clear. If you decrease your insulin levels, you'll lose weight (Fung, 2016).

One theorized mechanism by which insulin makes you fat states the following: insulin causes a chain of events that turns glucose into glycogen. Glycogen is stored in our liver, but its storage capacity is limited. Once our glycogen storage capacity reaches its limit, excess carbohydrates or blood sugars are then transformed and stored as fat in a process called lipogenesis.

Cortisol: The Energy Releasing Hormone

Cortisol is known as the stress hormone, and we already talked about its effects on the microbiome. This hormone makes you gain weight; it increases your glucose, which consequently increases your insulin levels.

We can imagine why cortisol would increase your blood sugar: it's because we release it when we must overcome an obstacle associated with the fight or flight response. When we need to get something done, like meeting a deadline, getting up for work, or defending ourselves from a predator, we should be alert and have energy at our disposal to do so. We wouldn't want to feel groggy or tired when we're in a dire situation. This is why cortisol increases our blood sugar so that we can meet the possible demands for energy we may come across. We would definitely need access to this energy if we were running late for a plane trip or trying to fend for our lives.

Our first energy source is glucose. Glucose is used by all the cells in our bodies to carry out their different functions. When our blood sugar levels decrease, our liver releases the glycogen it has stored in our liver to boost our glucose levels once more. This happens about 4 to 8 hours after we eat, depending on how resistant our body is to insulin and how high the insulin levels remain after eating.

This is why exercise is so good. Exercise is a way in which we can release cortisol, and we can cause ourselves stress. The good part is that we only release cortisol for a short period of time, and we actually burn the energy we make available. If we burn through our blood sugar levels first, then we begin to burn the glycogen we have stored.

When we're stressed, we're asking our body for more energy without putting it to use. If we ask our body for energy, we should use it. Through exercise, we ask for energy, and we use it. This allows us to tap into other sources of energy. We talked about how insulin stores glucose as glycogen in the liver; when we exercise, we're tapping into our glycogen storage, assuming that the exercise is intense enough to decrease your blood sugar levels. Once your glycogen is depleted in your liver, your body begins to tap into fat as a fuel source and turns fat into blood sugar for your cells to use. This is why cortisol can be useful for weight loss when we release it in short bursts.

These bursts of cortisol are what the body is designed for (Fung, 2016). Chronic stress acts quite differently; it makes energy available by increasing our blood sugar levels, even if there is no activity present in which we can use up the energy we have made available. This is why worrying or using your imagination to think about stressful situations excessively (anxious behaviors) can be so detrimental to your body weight and hormonal equilibrium. Obesity is only a hormonal imbalance after all.

Sleep deprivation raises your cortisol levels, consequently increasing your insulin levels and helping you gain weight. Fung (2016) mentions that sleeping less than 7 hours is when you start to be more likely to gain weight. We will talk a lot more about sleep deprivation in a later chapter.

Chronic stress makes our body insulin resistant, which only increases the amount of insulin our body needs to produce in order to store energy. (Fung, 2016).

Resistance, in the general sense, refers to our cells' ability to adapt. Suppose our body has continuously high levels of insulin throughout the day. In that case, it will try to find some balance and adjust to the increased levels of insulin by making our cells less sensitive to the hormone's presence. It's a defense mechanism. If your cells are less sensitive to insulin, it will take more insulin to satisfy your cells' demand for energy. Insulin opens a door for energy/glucose to get into the cells (Fung, 2016).

This idea of developing resistance is what the principle of vaccination is based on. We expose ourselves to a small amount of a pathogen to develop a certain tolerance to it, in the same way that some bacteria can develop resistance to antibiotics, which makes us have to use more antibiotics, unfortunately, leading to more antibiotic resistant pathogens.

Tolerance to chemicals is our body's defense mechanism. This is the same type of phenomenon that we may observe in substance addiction. An alcoholic's cells adapt to the increasingly high amount of dopamine in the body by making the person less sensitive to this "feel good" hormone. If somebody makes themselves less sensitive to the hormone that is supposed to make them feel happy, it means that they'll have a more challenging time feeling joy from life's simple pleasures.

Those small wins that we experience from seeing our loved ones or after a successful work week just become dull. They become dull in comparison to the joy we feel when we drink, because drinking releases much higher levels of dopamine than gazing at a sunset, for example.

To avoid antibiotic resistant pathogens, we need to cut down the amount of antibiotics we use. In this same sense, we must decrease the amount of insulin we expose our cells to. Insulin resistance is built up over time, and once you're insulin resistant, your insulin levels stay high. It's a self-sustaining cycle.

You can think of it this way; stress can spike your insulin just like eating can. Chronic stress is much like continuous snacking in the sense that it keeps your body's insulin levels high throughout the day. As we've seen, excessive insulin levels lead to insulin resistance, which causes us to store more fat than we usually would, since our cells become less sensitive to the hormone.

Famine & Feasting

Our eating schedule has changed since the 1970s. We've gone from eating three meals a day to accepting the idea that eating more often can actually help your metabolism (Fung, 2016). Now we've switched to eating six times a day on average.

Our eating schedule is the second factor that is involved in an increased resistance to insulin. Insulin is supposed to be released in a burst during the time we eat in order to absorb the energy that is being ingested. After eating, we're supposed to allow our insulin levels to drop down so that our body doesn't get accustomed to excessively high levels of insulin.

That's precisely the problem with snacking. If you eat every 2.5 hours or so, you won't allow your body's insulin levels to drop, which means that you will never use up any of the energy you have stored up as glycogen or fat while making your cells resistant to insulin. This is the science behind the intermittent fasting approaches that you may have heard about. The idea is to create a smaller eating window of about 8 hours in which you will consume all the calories you would normally consume; therefore, spiking your insulin levels.

Afterward, you will allow your body to decrease its insulin levels for the remaining 16 hours of the day. These 16 hours take your sleeping hours into account, so you would only really be cutting some eating time during the morning, evening, or both. It's your choice!

Your body will then have the time to decrease your blood sugar levels allowing you to tap into the glycogen that is stored in your liver and, once that's depleted, you can finally start to turn excess fat into a fuel source. If you exercise while you're in your fasted state, cortisol will ask your liver for energy and expedite the fat burning process.

Intermittent fasting is just about creating an eating schedule. You can start with a 12/12 window for the first week. Then on week two, you can switch to the 16/8 hour eating schedule. Ideally, make your last meal 3 hours before you sleep if you like to eat late at night. You can do this for about two weeks per month to begin with. There are more aggressive approaches, such as a 48 hour extended fast and water fasts. These other fasts have a lot of science backing them up as well, but they're also a lot more difficult to fit into everybody's lifestyle. This is why, for the time being, I would recommend setting up an eating schedule instead.

There's quite a vast amount of literature about the effects intermittent fasting has on your body, which goes beyond just balancing out your insulin levels. One of the benefits should not come as a surprise. If you think about it, fasting is a great way to increase your self-control. It's a way to stop acting on all your impulses, and it's a way to liberate ourselves from our body's every desire. It's a form of discipline. If you're able to overcome one of your body's most fundamental needs, hunger, it may become easier for you to make yourself clean your house when you're feeling tired, for example.

Self-control is a psychological benefit from fasting, but there are quite a few physiological effects as well. The physiological effects of fasting, which I'm about to discuss, begin after 8 hours of eating your last meal. These 8 hours I mention could be reduced if you exercise while you're in a fasted state since it would speed up the time in which you use up your stored energy. This is because by that time, most people would have already used up all their blood sugar, and the glycogen stored in their liver as fuel, so we begin to tap into a cleaner source of energy that is used by taking our fat and converting it into ketones.

Ketones are a cleaner energy source because they produce fewer free radicals than the energy we use from glucose. In later chapters, we'll discuss what free radicals are. Our body does this because it enters survival mode, and it's our body's way of preventing the loss of muscle mass. We can't live on ketones alone either, glucose is necessary, but with intermittent fasting, we can balance between these fuel sources.

Fasting not only changes our energy source, but it also stimulates the production of a set of proteins called brain derived neurotrophic factors. These proteins are involved in the growth of new brain cells and stimulating them to create new connections between them. Longer fasts see a larger increase in these proteins. The longest recommendable fast at the current time is 48 hours. There are some costs related to this fast because we begin to lose muscle mass after the third day. This is why I recommend intermittent fasting instead. It's a safe way in which anybody can reap the benefits of having a healthy eating schedule (Mattson, et. al., 2018).

The goal of fasting is triggering our body's defense mechanisms, making it change fuel sources for some periods in our day. We don't need to run on sugars all day, every day. This is not how our bodies have worked historically. It makes sense that our body would place us in a state where our brain becomes more alert and ready to learn from the environment. If we haven't eaten for a while, it would be adaptive for us to be prepared to hunt and be in an alert state, so that we can find more food and survive.

Obesity & Microbiota

There's contradictory evidence as far as our microbiome's role in obesity goes. Research on mice was carried out, and lean mice were turned into obese mice and vice-versa through the alteration of their microbiome. The microbiome was altered by transplanting the obese mice's fecal matter into the lean mices gut. These results were not successfully reproduced in humans, though (Sanmiguel, Gupta, & Mayer, 2015). Studies on twin humans also yielded conflicting results. There may be a relationship between our microbiome and obesity, but we haven't found it yet.

The yeasts or fungi that we have talked about can give us one clue to a possible relationship, though. It's theorized that our microbiota can influence our food preferences by interacting with our central nervous system through the vagus nerve. The vagus nerve is the link between the brain and the gut.

Most of the hormones that are key to our moods are located in the gut, so it would make sense that microorganisms could manipulate our likes and dislikes. In fact, research shows that the overpopulation of certain microbiota can alter the constitution of our taste buds to meet their own needs (Sanmiguel, Gupta, & Mayer, 2015).

Our vagus nerve is responsible for stimulating our appetite. In other words, if our vagus nerve is unable to relay information to our brain, we will lose weight (Alcock, et. al., 2014). Alternatively, overstimulation of this nerve will make you hungry more often, and our gut microbes are designed to be able to interact with our vagus nerve. This means that in some cases of bacterial overgrowth, some organisms could possibly overstimulate our vagus nerve, consequently giving us a sweet tooth or simply increasing our appetite. Much work must still be done in this field however.

As I said, research regarding the relationship between the microbiome, our eating behaviors, and obesity is still largely unknown. For the time being, it's safer to stick to the hormone balancing methods we've discussed.

Setting up an eating schedule is one of the more essential parts of lowering your insulin levels. The second factor is avoiding processed carbohydrates and sugars and keeping sugar at less than 25 grams per day. Processed foods are unrecognizable to our body's enzymes, which makes them difficult to digest. We should avoid most processed foods, like potato chips. Finally, we want to use cortisol to our advantage and understand how stress and exercise play roles in our body's hormonal balance. Like Fung (2016) states, obesity is a hormonal imbalance, not a moral failing.

In the following chapter, we will be looking to understand more about the different mechanisms through which our gut and brain communicate with each other. We've mentioned one so far: the vagus nerve. In addition, we'll look at how the link between our gut and our brain could be involved in mental health.

CHAPTER 06
MENTAL HEALTH

The gut is now known by many as the second brain. This is because a large amount of neurons relevant to our behavior and moods are also located in our enteric nervous system. Our enteric nervous system is made of connections between nerve cells and enterocytes situated all along our intestinal lining.

These enterocytes have sensors that allows them to detect chemical, mechanical, and thermal changes in their environment. They communicate these changes to the nerve cells that they're connected to by sending electrochemical messages. Microbiota and their metabolites can stimulate these enterocytes and send messages to the nerve cells attached to them. The neurons or nerve cells linked to the enterocytes are part of a pathway of electrochemical information called the vagus nerve.

The vagus nerve is a bidirectional information duct between the brainstem and our enteric nervous system. Communication via this duct takes only a few seconds. This means that the food we ingest can alter our brain states rather quickly (Sharon et. al., 2016).

One of the hormones used to communicate with our brain is serotonin; 95% of the serotonin in our body is produced in our gut (Sharon et. al., 2016). Like we've discussed, serotonin is involved in many complex mechanisms, such as sleep, sexual desire, and mood. A lack of serotonin is thought to be correlated with depressive and sleep disorders.

Serotonin is produced from compounds that we receive through our diet. In fact, 60% of the serotonin produced in our gut is produced due to microbial stimulation (Sharon et. al., 2016). The microbiota in our gut can inhibit or stimulate serotonin production.

Our microbiota produces and stores most of our mood-regulating hormones, so it's safe to believe they must play a large role in our emotional/hormonal equilibrium.

We could even hypothesize that some pathogens may be able to manipulate our cravings and behaviors to some degree. If we give the pathogens what they want, they could possibly stimulate the production of serotonin and dopamine, so we feel good and rewarded for doing their bidding. The scenario that comes to mind would be our consumption of certain sugars. Studies have shown differences in the microbiome of people with a sweet tooth (Chao et. al, 2017). Perhaps these people's reward centers are being manipulated by their microbiota. The microbes can inhibit the release and production of these neurotransmitters, making us feel down if we don't get them what they want. These are all just possible ideas about the interactions that might occur in the gut-brain axis.

Depression & Cortisol

We're going to use depression as an example of how our microbiome is involved in our emotional states and mental health. However, research links the microbiome to neurodegenerative diseases such as Alzheimer's and Parkinson's disease. For illustration purposes, we're going to focus on depression, especially since depression is a very relevant condition in our era, and it often coexists with bacterial dysbiosis, obesity, IBS, and sleep disorders.

Suicide rates and depression are on a steady rise in our modern era (Planap & Hest, 2019; SAMHSA, 2013; Stossel, 2013). It's quite odd because we're living in the age of comfort and technology. You would think people would feel connected and less lonely because of the internet, or people would be more relaxed with the amount of convenience and comfort at our disposal. We no longer have to hunt for our food. Instead, we can just order our groceries and have them delivered to our doorstep.

Depression is most often born out of sadness, and sadness is usually linked to a loss of some sort. In loneliness, it would be a loss of meaningful connections, for example. There is a fundamental difference between sadness and depression because it has to do with our resilience and how we deal with the stress of loss. The experience of loss brings about sadness as a means to tell us that we should make amendments. It's a way we're able to know that what we lost mattered to us, so the stress this experience brings about is supposed to make us want to do something about it. Its purpose is to fix a situation or look to regain what was lost. This is sadness's reparative function.

Depression, on the other hand, is associated with a black and white way of thinking. A depressed individual is unable to see past their situation of pain and suffering. We only see the bad and have forgotten all the good in our lives. Depression can lead to suicide, mainly because of this black and white way of seeing the world. When you don't believe that things will be okay again, and focus only on the bad, you lose hope. It's okay to feel sad, but a sad person experiences the painful sensations of their emotion while remembering all the good in life while also keeping in mind that things will be okay once again.

Disturbances in bodily cortisol levels have been noticed in individuals suffering from depression. Some depressed people have shown irregularly high cortisol levels in the morning while others display them at night; these could be signs of different types of depression, but more research is still required to determine this fact.

It's known that increased cortisol levels exist in individuals suffering from depressive disorders, but it's unknown if cortisol is the cause or a symptom. What is known is that excessive exposure to cortisol can reduce the amount of connections between the neurons in our brain, while also decreasing the amount of new neurons that are born. These effects may explain why people's perception of their world becomes limited during depressive states; thought patterns become very rigid. Depressed people are unable to see the actual OPTIONS they have in life. A sort of tunnel vision is experienced during depressive states, like a cognitive nearsightedness that may be caused by cortisol's disruptions in the processes involved in our perception of reality.

Leaky Gut & Depression

Our understanding of depression has drastically changed since we've gained a better understanding of the enteric nervous system. Depression was thought to be born from a lack of certain neurotransmitters such as dopamine and serotonin; this theory is how antidepressants were born. Now we've begun to understand that there are much more complex interactions and that the decreased production of these neurotransmitters is only one factor involved in depression.

We've talked about how chronically high cortisol levels in our body can deteriorate the state of our intestinal lining and even cause dysbiosis. Cortisol disturbances are also noticed to play a role in major depressive and anxiety disorders. Like with insulin, persistently high cortisol levels can make our cortisol receptors resistant to the hormone, making our body increase our cortisol levels.

IBD and depression commonly coexist and reinforce each other. We've talked about how depression and the chronic stress derived from pain can damage our intestinal wall, but now we want to talk about how IBD can cause and reinforce depression. Leaky gut syndrome (LGS) is a term used to describe an excessively permeable intestinal wall. When our intestinal wall is overly permeable, it begins to let toxic waste and microorganisms into our body.

Leaky gut is mainly caused by the cytokines produced through excessive activation of the sympathetic nervous system, releasing high cortisol levels. Corrosive components in our diet, such as emulsifiers, can damage our intestinal lining directly. High sugar intake also damages our intestinal lining indirectly through dysbiosis. This is because our commensal bacteria serve as a bacterial barrier that protects our intestinal lining; not having enough communities of them on our walls will also lead to a leaky gut.

Once particles and microorganisms breach our intestinal lining, they're able to travel to different organs and cells in our body through the bloodstream or interact with our nervous system through the vagus nerve. It's theorized that this is why IBD coexists with depression and autoimmune diseases, such as arthritis. In arthritis, the toxins are able to lodge themselves in our joints and cause an inflammatory response by our immune system as it tries to keep them out. In this same way, our central nervous system's glial cells fire inflammatory responses as well.

Glial cells are our nervous system's autoimmune components. They're the cells that protect our brain from possible pathogenic colonization. Our glial cells can save our life through inflammation; this is how they keep toxins out of our brain and central nervous system. However, continuously having these glial cells activated has profound effects on our brain chemistry and composition. There's a whole body of psychiatric literature about the interaction of hyperactive glial cells and depression, although this interaction isn't new (Ludzki, Leszek & Maes, 2020). What is newly added knowledge to our scientific body of research is the interaction between leaky gut and our glial cells.

There are many types of glial cells, and each of those glial cells has their specific functions. They also play specific roles in depression. Microglia, for example, play a large role in synaptic pruning. Synaptic pruning is when our brain cuts off connections between neurons. Our brain uses synaptic pruning as a means of being efficient. If we don't use certain connections, there's no need to keep them. For example, if you stop practicing the violin for about 30 years, perhaps the connections that were used for certain violin notes may be put to better use elsewhere.

Our microglia are involved in synaptic pruning, so could it be that over activating these cells could lead to unnecessary loss of synaptic connections? Our microglia are activated by the toxins released from our gut. This is just one example of a possible way in which overactive glial cells could damage our brain cells. We did mention that there's a loss of synaptic connections in individuals with depression; it was shown to be related to the excessive presence of cortisol, but it's possible that overactivation of our glial cells could reinforce this same effect.

If toxins are continuously seeping through our leaky gut and forcing our glial cells to cause inflammation, our glial cells will eventually get worn out or disfigured in different ways. We're pretty much turning our defenses against ourselves. The implications of these findings mean that we need to have a more holistic approach to mental health. Holistic comes from the word "whole," and it refers to seeing the whole picture and taking into consideration all the interactions between the different parts in the picture.

Mental health was thought to be solely a disease of the brain or soul, but we've come very far from those times, and now we understand that the microbes in our gut and the enteric nervous system itself require a great deal of attention.

As we've seen, stress and cortisol still plays a large role in all of these different illnesses, so I'm going to give you another way to reduce stress. These methods are referred to as breathwork, meditation, and mindfulness training. Breathwork is quite interesting. It's one of the only ways in which we can control our autonomic nervous system. When we inhale, we're activating the sympathetic nervous system that stimulates cortisol secretion. When we exhale, we're activating the parasympathetic nervous system, which we mentioned was associated with regeneration and healing.

The following exercise is called diaphragmatic breathing, and it's going to be the first step in reducing your resting cortisol levels.

Breathwork Exercise

Sit down or stand up in a relaxed position, either way is fine. If you prefer to do your breathwork standing, I would recommend tai chi or yoga, which are art forms that incorporate breathwork while moving.

Inhale for 4 seconds, then **hold** your breath for 4 seconds. When you reach your maximum air capacity, try to inhale a bit more, so that your diaphragm dilates slightly. **Afterward**, exhale for 4 seconds, and hold the void for 4 seconds. **Repeat this process** 3 to 4 times until you enter a relaxed state of mind.

You can extend the time periods, particularly when you hold your breath. You may hold your breath as long as you please; in fact, I recommend you push your limits with this exercise.

Once you've entered a relaxed state of mind, you will move into mindfulness meditation. This type of meditation is designed to slow down the racing thoughts that come to your mind and slow down your reactions to them. The idea behind this is to help you stop being over-identified with your thoughts, emotions, and behaviors.

When you're overidentifying with your thoughts and behaviors, you tend to live out life in a reactive way and not a proactive way. This is one reason we want to bring our typically automatic breathing process into awareness. It's the first unconscious process that we'll make conscious. An example of being overidentified with your actions is noticed in the difference between shame and guilt. Let's say you make a mistake since all of us make mistakes. Guilt is a way we tell ourselves we're not acting in alignment with our values and that we should make some changes. Shame, on the other hand, is when we believe we ARE our mistakes. It's our inability to separate ourselves from our thoughts, emotions, and actions. When you're ashamed, you feel like there's something inherently wrong about you. You ARE much more than the time you yelled at your loved one, the time you forgot the keys in the car, or the time you lost your job.

Shame is a driving factor of different pain-causing stress responses. It fuels excessive anger and depression. This is just one example of how creating space between you and your emotions, thoughts, and actions can help in the way you react to them.

The following exercise aims to create space between yourself and your thoughts, emotions, and behaviors. You will take an impartial, non-judgemental observer role in relation to yourself.

Mindfulness Meditation Practice

Once you're done with the breathing exercise I gave you, you can continue sitting or lying down. Music and olfactory stimulation are valid options as well.

Close your eyes. Now, gently **stop creating new thoughts and stop moving;** do this for **5 minutes** at first. Later on, you can increase it to 10 minutes and even 30 minutes.

As you stop creating thoughts, you will notice that thoughts and emotions will come to you spontaneously, even if you're not asking for them. Just observe them, and understand that this happens throughout the whole day. This is how you'll come to realize that you ARE not your thoughts since they're coming to you even without you creating them.

You may ask those thoughts why they've come to you at that specific time if you please.

If awareness was a muscle, this is the exercise you use to strengthen it. It allows you to be more aware of the different thoughts that race into you. Little by little, you will train yourself to be more self-aware in your daily routine. Consequently, you will gain the ability to choose how you want to react to different stressful situations, instead of acting out your pre-conditioned patterns.

Psychobiotics

Psychobiotics is the name proposed for probiotics that are neurologically active. They stimulate the production of or produce psychoactive substances, which could be beneficial to our mental health. The mechanisms by which they do this are still under investigation. One theory is worth mentioning is the one which refers to the production of gaba amino butyric acid (GABA).

It's known that lactobacillus and bifidobacterium genera are associated with an increased level of GABA. So the idea is that psychobiotics should be able to influence our response to stress through the production of GABA and its interactions with our amygdala (Snigdha & Debapriya, 2017).

Our amygdala is an evolutionarily primitive part of our brain that is associated with our fear/anxiety and stress responses. Basic emotions that we need for our survival as a species, such as fear or anxiety (so we could run away from danger) and anger (so we could fight off a predator) are born from the systems of neurons either within the amygdala or directly connected to it.

GABA is an inhibiting neurotransmitter, which means it deactivates whatever neuron it comes across. There are neurons connected to our amygdala which releases GABA. GABA is supposed to regulate our fear, anger, and stress responses by acting on the amygdala. When GABA is released, we're supposed to be able to bounce back from our sensations of stress. Our ability to inhibit or regulate our emotions comes from the messages GABA is able to relay.

Anxiety comes from an overactive amygdala causing overactive fear circuits to fire. Our amygdala can stimulate the production of cortisol when it's activated, so an overactive amygdala means excessive cortisol levels as well.

Substances such as alcohol and cannabis act upon our GABA receptors. This is why we feel sedated when we consume these substances. They stimulate GABA release in large amounts, which deactivates our amygdala, consequently reducing our anxiety. The issue is that just like with any other chemical; our cells will eventually become resistant to it. Not only this, but releasing extremely high GABA amounts through drug use will ultimately deplete your GABA storage.

This is particularly why depressants, such as cannabis and alcohol, can be detrimental to emotional regulation. If you don't have enough GABA to inhibit your anger or fear, or your neurons have become resistant to it, you won't be able to manage the ups and downs we all experience. When you feel happy, you will feel really happy to the point where you become manic, and when you feel sad, you will become depressed instead of just sad. Bipolar personality disorder or manic depression can be the outcome of damaged GABA systems.

In this same sense, anger is really difficult to inhibit without a properly functioning GABA system. This may be why alcohol is often involved with incidences of violent behaviors.

Psychobiotics proposes an alternative means to reduce anxiety and regulate your emotions by increasing the amount of GABA that is produced by Lactobacillus and Bifidobacterium genera. There are other natural supplements that increase the efficiency in which GABA is transported, though. This is just a theory for the time being. Until more clinical research is carried out, these known methods for increasing GABA efficiency are recommended.

There are two more theories regarding how psychobiotics could influence our moods and behavior. We've already talked about the other two theories extensively, though. The first one is that leaky gut is the mechanism by which our glial cells are overactivated, producing excessive inflammatory responses. The overactivation of our immune system is thought to bring about inflammation and fatigue, which causes the mutation or deformation of the cells affected. The second theory is about the hormonal balance of serotonin, dopamine, and cortisol. We've covered this theory in great detail as well.

We haven't reached the point of being able to target particular mental illnesses with specific strains yet, so I'm not so sure how useful the term "psychobiotics" is right now. Until a product is released that stands the tests of science, we're better off just sticking to more conventional forms of treatment, while of course, keeping a healthy and diverse microbiome (Snigdha & Debapriya, 2017).

Next, we're going to be talking about how sleep ties into this whole situation. None of the different issues we've talked about are isolated in any way, which is why a holistic approach is imperative.

CHAPTER 07
ADEQUATE SLEEP

Like the passing of the seasons and the star patterns we use to tell time, our body is also ruled by cycles. The hormonal processes in our body follow a structured pattern throughout the day, called the circadian rhythm. The circadian rhythm governs our wakefulness cycles and our transitions into sleep, while our sleep stages describe the patterns and processes experienced during our slumber. We're going to be looking into how our microbiota influences these cycles.

Circadian Rhythm & Sleep Stages

The circadian rhythm is what people call their biological or internal clock. It's a 24-hour pattern that governs our sleep/wake cycles. One of the primary environmental cues that our brain is programmed to follow is light, particularly blue light that comes from the sun. This is why our internal clock is synchronized with the day and night cycles. Light does not create the cycle. We're already wired to have a 24-hour cycle; light only synchronizes our cycle.

Light triggers a chain of electrochemical impulses in our brain that leads to the propagation of hormonal messages throughout the body.

Our hormone levels are also synchronized with these cycles, such as in the morning, towards the end of our sleep cycles, and when our cortisol levels hit a peak. Cortisol and serotonin are released, so we wake up and transition into an alert state. Throughout the day, our cortisol levels continue to fluctuate. Cortisol's fluctuation is primarily based on how much blue light we receive through our retina. In the evening, cortisol drops to its lowest point, at which time our pineal gland secretes melatonin.

The pineal gland has photoreceptors just like our retina does, which allow it to sense when light is coming through. When light comes through, melatonin production is suppressed, and cortisol is released. When melatonin peaks, cortisol is suppressed. Cortisol wakes you up, and melatonin puts you to sleep. Once melatonin puts you to sleep, which can take up to 20 minutes, another set of cycles begin.

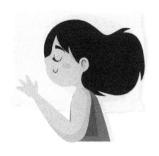

Sleep Stages:

Stage 1 NREM (non-rapid eye movement) 1

Stage 2 NREM (non-rapid eye movement) 2

Stage 3 NREM 3: slow-wave sleep (SWS)

Stage 4 REM (rapid eye movement)

These stages work in 90-minute cycles; in the first cycle, REM sleep is not experienced. Sleep stages are characterized by the type of brain waves we emit throughout each of the stages. In those 20 minutes, while we're going to sleep, we're moving from alpha and beta waves, which are associated with wakefulness into theta waves. Theta waves occur in those moments that you're in between being asleep and awake. This is called a hypnagogic state; people have reported hallucinations, feelings of falling, and even muscle jerks during this phase. Theta waves are also present in meditative states, which is why people report having visions while practicing meditation. This whole transitional phase of sleep is called stage 1 sleep of the non-rapid eye movement (NREM) stage.

As you transition from NREM 1 to NREM 2, theta waves increase, and now sleep spindles appear. Sleep spindles are short bursts of brain activity that are associated with learning and memory. Sleep spindles are also hypothesized to allow us to ignore external stimuli; they act as a way of suppressing sounds and sensations while we sleep so that we stay asleep. This is why it's more difficult to wake somebody up in this second stage of sleep.

NREM 3 is called slow-wave sleep (SWS) because we move from theta to delta waves. At this point, it's very challenging to wake somebody up. This type of sleep is deep, and there isn't much dream activity at this point. SWS is characterized by an increased activation of the parasympathetic nervous system. This is where regenerative physiological processes take place. These brain waves stimulate the release of the human growth hormone (HGH), called somatotropin. The HGH's function is to make nutrients more available in your body for your muscle and skeletal cells to have the energy or ATP. This is necessary for your body to create new proteins. This is when a large portion of our damaged tissues are repaired. HGH in our blood makes nutrients available by stimulating our body fat and liver.

Our adipose tissue is our body fat. HGH can stimulate this tissue, and it can be requested to break our fat into simpler molecules called fatty acids. These fatty acids can be used by our body's cells as a fuel source in order to heal our body. On the other hand, our liver is triggered to release blood sugar into the bloodstream by converting the glycogen it has stored into glucose. This is also done with the purpose of fueling the cells implicated in our body's reparative processes.

SWS makes it so our body has more nutrients available to it through the release of HGH. HGH also makes our cells able to receive more nutrients by increasing their uptake. This is why sleep is so important on a physical level.

REM sleep is the next stage; we experience this type of sleep more towards the end of the night, closer to when we're about to wake up. The REM sleep's brain wave patterns are similar to those found in wakeful states of mind, which is why our body paralyzes our muscles, so that we don't hurt ourselves through the increased brain activity. This increased brain activity is the reason why REM sleep displays the largest amount of dream content.

Dreams and REM sleep are crucial to our cognitive processes and the strengthening of our neural pathways. In this stage of sleep, our sympathetic nervous system is activated, and with it comes an increase in our cortisol levels. Cortisol plays a large role in the process of dream formation through our memory structures. There are two types of memories that are governed by the different systems of neurons in our brain. The first type is called episodic memory. This type of memory is related to time and space-specific information, and it allows us to recall events with their accurate times and places. Semantic memory, on the other hand, refers to the memory of concepts and categories. Being able to place a banana in the fruit category is an example of semantic memory.

During REM sleep, the increased levels of cortisol shut down our episodic memory while leaving our semantic memory untouched (Payne & Nadel, 2002). This is what causes the fragmented aspect of dreams reported during REM sleep. You may have a dream of sitting at an ice cream parlor with your boss who, in your dream, was your father at the same time, while a talking octopus took your order. This combination of categories and concepts is possible when we remove episodic memory from the equation.

The deconstruction of categories during REM sleep allows us to recombine unrelated ideas and concepts in order to give birth to new ideas. This is one way creativity occurs; we create new ideas through mixing concepts during this stage of sleep. This process also integrates what we learned throughout the day into our long-term memories by combining new experiences with old ones. The increased brain activity looks to reinforce our neural pathways.

As you can see, sleep is implicated in our regenerative processes, but also in the consolidation of new information and creativity. It's imperative that we must get adequate sleep.

Microbiome & Sleep

Just like humans, microorganisms have circadian rhythms. In fact, that's how the circadian rhythm was discovered; through an increase of eukaryotes' population size during specific times of the day, which was observed in plants (Li, Hao, & Zhang, 2018).

Clock genes have a direct connection with our microbiota. Studies have shown a correlation between our microbiota and how clock genes are expressed (Li, Hao, & Zhang, 2018). Clock genes are the specific genetic material in charge of producing the proteins required to regulate our circadian rhythms. Our microorganisms can cause a mutation in our clock genes and make them hyperactivate the glands that release cortisol. Consequently, it disrupts our sleep patterns and makes us more likely to develop depressive symptoms, IBS, and increasingly high insulin resistance levels.

This hyperactivation of our cortisol releasing system goes back and reduces our microbial biodiversity, causing dysbiosis and eventually, a leaky gut. Having a leaky gut weakens our immune system by over activating it and alters our hormonal balance making us more susceptible to diseases and stress. Our ability to cope with life's stressors diminishes, since the increased resting cortisol levels in our body make it hard to bounce back from a difficult experience (Li, Hao, & Zhang, 2018). The widespread inflammation caused by a leaky gut is itself linked to sleeping disorders and mental illness.

Furthermore, serotonin is associated with the occurrence of REM sleep and the appearance of depressive symptoms (Li, Hao, & Zhang, 2018). Most serotonin production is stimulated by our microbiota. Without serotonin, the amount of REM sleep we get is diminished as well.

Studies have shown that GABA helps prevent insomnia and depression. As previously mentioned, Lactobacillus and Bifidobacterium genera are known to produce GABA, so it may be in our best interest to tilt the scale in their favor and give them the fiber-rich foods they desire (Li, Hao, & Zhang, 2018).

The mutually reinforcing relationship our microbiota shares with our sleep disorders is clear. Although, there's much to be learned about the mechanisms as to how this is occurring. For now, our best bet would be to approach this issue holistically and tackle all the factors as a whole.

Creating Good Sleeping Habits

Here are a few tips using the scientific data we just went over. These will be useful whether you're having trouble falling asleep, staying asleep, or simply feeling sluggish and tired throughout the day. Remember, it's not just about the quantity of sleep, but the quality of sleep is also imperative.

Daylight is going to be driving our energy levels and conditioning our bodies. If we're exposed to sunlight on a regular basis, our body will remain synchronized, and eventually, it will be programmed to know when it's supposed to release cortisol and how much to release. To maintain adequate energy levels throughout the day, you want to follow a regular and consistent sleep schedule, so you don't throw your body off course.

If you have trouble falling asleep, it's because you're activating your sympathetic nervous system late at night and releasing too much cortisol, which will suppress your melatonin production. You may be doing this by looking at screens before bed and not using night-time mode. The screens on our phones and computers emit blue light, much like the sun, tricking our pineal gland into thinking it's still daytime. Ideally, you want to refrain from looking at screens at least one hour before going to bed. If this isn't possible, use night-time mode which should make your screen look a dark orange color.

Overstimulating work, such as homework or any challenging tasks, should be avoided in the last hour before sleep. Challenging tasks release cortisol, acetylcholine, and dopamine, making you alert, focused, and aroused, respectively. One especially detrimental activity for sleep is playing video games. They combine blue light with challenging tasks, which is perfect for keeping you alert and awake.

Meditation, as you try to go to sleep, is recommended since this activity itself creates theta waves. Theta waves are characteristics of our first two sleep stages. My recommendation would be to place a limit on how long you're allowed to reflect upon your life and day before bed. Give yourself about 5 minutes or 10 if you wish, but then stop creating new thoughts and practice clearing your mind. The style of meditation you want to use is of your choosing.

If you're still having trouble falling asleep and you just lie there tossing and turning, you can get up and stretch gently. Afterwards, you can engage in a light activity, such as reading, until you become sleepy once more. Just make sure you're using an actual book instead of an electronic device.

A melatonin supplement can help you set up your sleep schedule. These are non-addictive and non-invasive, and you won't feel tired the next day. As studies have recently shown, the best part is that melatonin supplements that include vitamin B6 can help increase our microbiome's biodiversity (Li, Hao, & Zhang, 2018).

Another trick you may want to try is taking a cold shower before you go to bed, preferably in that last hour, when you shouldn't be engaging in any other activities anyway. A cold shower is best, but a warm shower works fine as well since both will reduce your body temperature. Your circadian rhythm also regulates your body temperature throughout the day and, when it's bedtime, your body temperature is supposed to drop. So dropping your body temperature intentionally is a way of tricking your body into thinking it's time to sleep.

People think that using alcohol or cannabis helps them sleep, but these depressants sedate you, and there's a difference between being sedated and sleeping. Your sleep stages are disrupted particularly your SWS and REM stages. So you may sleep the hours necessary, but the following day you will still feel tired because you didn't reap the benefits from these critical sleep stages.

Finally, we can condition our brain to make associations, just like you can train a dog to learn a new trick. Use your bed to only sleep. Don't allow your brain to associate your bed with watching tv or playing video games. Using your bed as an environmental cue is a simple but necessary practice.

If you're still feeling sleepy throughout the day, even after implementing these practices, you may want to try to let some sunshine hit you in the morning. Going out in the sun will make your retina signal the release of cortisol while conditioning you to have energy at that time of the day. A cold shower in the morning can also help you get a head start on your day.

Conditioning our brain to have a consistent sleep schedule is very important. If you're not able to go to bed at the recommended time, which is 10 pm, then at least go to bed at the same time every night to help your body adjust its circadian rhythm.

Generally, from 10 pm till 2 am is when most of our HGH is released, so we don't want to miss this window. As I said before, our body is always ready to adapt, so if you need to shift your sleeping schedule to a later time, you have to make sure to be consistent with your body in order to condition it properly.

As you can see, sleep is imperative with its physiologically restorative properties and with how it helps us in our learning processes. However, we need to make sure we have an adequate amount of energy for our body to follow through with these vital restorative processes.

CHAPTER 08
EATING ENOUGH FOR YOUR BODY

As you can see, hormonal messages that are constantly sent throughout your body are responsible for keeping you motivated, focused, alert, and, when the time finally comes, relaxed. Our body makes sure we have the energy we need to survive in our fast-paced social environments, so we need to make sure our body has what it needs to make this possible.

When you wake up, you get out of bed because your body makes nutrients available through an increase in cortisol. Stress at a healthy level keeps us alert and ready for action. I don't want you to get the wrong impression by thinking that cortisol is bad. Without cortisol, getting out of our comfy bed would be nearly impossible.

We need to help our body keep its equilibrium by giving it the energy it requires to do its job. We'll discuss in this chapter why eating less and restrictive diets are not the cure-all solutions they've been made out to be. Since our body has a tendency to adapt and maintain an equilibrium through its homeostatic tendencies, eating less will cause our body to adapt to the lower amount of energy that is being introduced to the system.

We've discussed how a calorie is not a calorie; what this also implies is that there are many fuel sources we can draw from. It's known that we can use any of the macronutrients we consume, such as carbohydrates, proteins, or fats as fuel sources. Even the sugar we get from soft drinks or cheesecake can be used as a fuel source since it contains very high caloric values. Oxidative damage or oxidative stress is the reason we can consider some fuel sources cleaner than others.

While we're in pursuit of getting enough energy for our body, we may also want to make sure we're getting the cleanest energy we can get as well.

The Secrets To Improve Bloating, Digestion, Anxiety And Fat Loss

The "Eat Less" Myth

A common belief that many of us hold is that if you want to lose weight or be healthier, you simply need to reduce the size of your meal and the number of calories you're ingesting on a daily basis. It would make sense since the idea is that we gain weight because fewer calories are being spent as opposed to how many are consumed. The equation is intuitive—you would think that if you reduce the number of incoming calories, but continue to exercise in the same way, you will lose weight.

Our body has a tendency to adapt, however, so when we cut down the number of calories that we're ingesting, our body also decreases the number of calories or energy it spends (Fung, 2016). This means that fewer calories in means fewer calories out. This is why people don't just grow increasingly thin when they reduce their calorie intake. At first, you may lose weight, but after a couple of weeks, your body will adjust to the new calorie count.

Restricting the amount of food you eat isn't even a good strategy for losing weight. When you drastically reduce the amount of calories you ingest on a daily basis, the amount of leptin you produce is also decreased. Leptin is the hormone in charge of feelings of satiety. If you don't feel satiated, you'll feel even more hungry, and you may tend to overeat when you do eat. This is your body's way of telling you that you're not eating enough for your body.

When you're overweight, your body's hormones will set your "normal weight" at the weight you're currently at. Weight is regulated through hormonal messages, so if you eat less, your body will think it's not getting enough energy to keep you at your "normal weight." Mechanisms will begin to get you back up to your normal weight. You will feel more hungry and will spend less energy in order to keep your normal weight (Fung, 2016).

Your set weight is determined by hormonal balance. In order to lose weight, the presence of insulin in your body and your insulin resistance needs to be targeted. So, eating less is somewhat futile, and your body will work against you if you do that.

If we reduce our caloric intake too much, our vital functions will be prioritized, while leaving other bodily functions as secondary. Functions such as the absorption of nutrients or the regenerative processes of your body, such as periods in women, might be suspended in order to keep essential functions flowing smoothly.

You can be malnourished and still be obese. Using empty calories as your fuel source is the real danger. Empty calories may spike your blood sugar and insulin but provide little nutritional value. Snacks and desserts, like cheesecake, soft drinks, and potato chips are not only empty calories, but they're much worse than that since they cause inflammation and oxidation. We're going to talk about why using these junk foods as fuel sources is detrimental.

Free Radicals & Antioxidants

Oxygen has a corrosive effect when it comes in contact with many molecules, including the cells in our body. This corrosive effect is called oxidation. Oxidation is theorized to be the primary mechanism by which cancer and aging occur. This is because oxidation is inevitable, as long as we continue to need oxygen to survive. Although oxidation is unavoidable, there are ways to speed up or slow down the process.

Free radicals in our body are usually made up of oxygen. These are the waste products released when we use certain foods as fuel sources. These waste products are released when we create energy by inserting blood sugar into our cells. Once the waste products are released, they can blend with other cells in our body, destroying them or simply altering their behavior.

Our cells must repair themselves after being damaged by the free radicals that blend with them. If we continuously damage our cells, eventually, they may make a mistake during the repair process. These failures in their regenerative processes can lead to a mutation.

The mutation of cells just means that the cells become abnormal. This mutation causes our cells to stop cooperating with other cells and start multiplying. This contagion of mutant cells is what people refer to as cancer.

In our case, the number of free radicals released in our body can be increased by the type of fuel source we use. You can use carbon-based energy to fuel society, or you can use cleaner, more sustainable methods. The amount of waste or free radicals that are released is increased when you use highly processed sugars as your main energy source.

Mitochondria are the engines within our body's cells that produce the energy of life. They do this by taking our blood sugar and turning it into ATP. When these engines become damaged through repetitive interactions with free radicals, their ability to produce energy decreases. In other words, using unclean energy sources—meaning foods high on the glycemic index—will eventually leave you with less energy to work with in the long run.

You can think of insulin as the key that opens the door to our cells. Insulin allows blood sugar to go inside our cells, where it can be turned into energy by our mitochondria. The issue is that if we have high blood sugar by consuming sugar itself, we'll have an excess level of it in our blood. When it's found in excess in our blood, it's free to interact with other molecules and eventually creates free radicals.

If it's not clear by now, we don't need refined sugars in our diet because they don't provide any sort of benefit. All the sugars you need can be obtained from healthy carbs contained in fruit and vegetables. Cutting sugar out of your life will not act as a cure-all solution for oxidation or inflammation, but it's definitely a great place to start.

Inflammation stimulates the production of more free radicals through an increase in macrophages. This is a complex topic, so our key takeaway here is that the aging process and all sorts of cancer are exacerbated by inflammation. We know inflammation is worsened by sugar and stress, so we can now draw a connection between stress, sugar, inflammation, cancer, and aging.

Antioxidants are surrounded by marketing hype, so by now, I'm sure you're familiarized with the term. Since our body naturally produces free radicals, it has also created a defense mechanism against them. This is what an antioxidant is; it's a molecule that stabilizes the free radical waste products and turns them into molecules that won't harm our cells.

There are enzymes in our body that are responsible for turning free radicals into stable molecules. The issue is that high insulin levels neutralize these enzymes, which is one of the mechanisms by which sugar increases the amount of free radicals present in our bloodstream.

Some superfoods can help tilt the battle against free radicals in your favor. Unfortunately, the term "superfood" does little to describe an item. It's just another tool that marketing campaigns use to catch your attention. Although the blueberry industry has funded a large portion of the research carried out around blueberries, there does seem to be some truth as far as their antioxidant properties go. I'm using blueberries as an example simply because there's a lot of literature and research around them; however, there are many other foods that can provide similar effects.

The pigment found in dark, colorful fruit such as blueberries can catch and blend with free radicals, ultimately defusing them. As some have said, you should "eat the rainbow," meaning that you should get as many different colored fruit and vegetables in your diet as possible. Different colored nutrients can blend with different kinds of free radicals. Again, the solution is not just increasing your intake of blueberries, although including blueberries in your diet is excellent.

Sometimes we lose sight of the fact that we simply need to have a balanced diet and lifestyle instead of looking for a way to cheat the system by finding a "superfood." That's how propaganda gets you. It sells you hope. It sells you the key to your life. Marketers tell us: "you don't need to put any work into yourself, I have a cure-all solution for you!".

Curcumin and turmeric are great options as far as fighting free radicals goes. What's so great about them is that they're spices, so they're flexible. You can put them in a wide variety of dishes. Some people even put a little bit of them in their smoothies.

Another trick is related to avocados. In general, avocados are very useful, they provide healthy fats, and their fiber to carb ratio is ideal. The avocado's seed, however, has antioxidant properties. It can be ground up into powder with a food processor or a spice grinder. Drying the seed first makes the process easier. You can mince it with a knife into very fine pieces if you don't have a grinder or a processor. The taste is much like other seeds and nuts, plus you can use it much like the spices we previously mentioned. You can try sprinkling some avocado powder on top of your salad or your sugar-free smoothies.

Speaking of healthy fats, these can be a cleaner source of energy in which fewer free radicals are created. Healthy fats can be looked at as unsaturated fats that don't solidify at room temperature. Avocado oil, coconut oil, olive oil, omega 3s, omega 6s, and dark chocolate are some examples of healthy fats. Coconut oil is actually a type of saturated fat that is good for you at certain doses.

The difference between a medicine and a poison is the dose. Too much of a good thing is still too much. Just because olive oil is good for you, it doesn't mean that you should shower all your meals in oil.

The avocado seed we spoke about previously has been used since ancient times to treat gastrointestinal diseases. The polyphenols present in the avocado seed seem to act as a prebiotic that stimulates our microbiome's biodiversity by creating an antagonistic environment for pathogens (Segovia et. al., 2018).

Having a diverse and healthy microbiome has also been correlated with our energy levels. Less inflammation means that our body is using less energy to fight itself. Inflammation uses energy since it's our immune system firing off. Constant inflammation puts our body to work, so chronic fatigue is a natural side-effect.

On the other hand, small intestine bacterial overgrowth (SIBO) will make us compete for nutrients with microorganisms who relocate in our small intestine from our colon. Malnourishment and a lack of energy are a consequence of this. Sugar also strengthens organisms with flagella who can swim upstream into our small intestine. This is just another reason why we need to watch our sugar to fiber ratio.

We must make sure that we're eating enough for our body, but we must also make sure we're using the right fuel sources. Free radicals are inevitable, but high blood sugar will increase the speed at which they damage our cells at a molecular level.

Eat a diverse amount of healthy fats, fiber, and different colored fruit and vegetables while managing your stress levels. In essence, exercise, sleeping well, and learning how to unwind and relax can all act as anti-aging antioxidants.

I want us to be extremely careful with the way we approach our health since corporations can take this very noble intention of wanting to love yourself and use it for their own materialistic gains.

CHAPTER 09
PARASITIC CORPORATIONS & PARASITIC MICROORGANISMS

Consumerism ties in directly with the state of our microbial biodiversity. In this chapter, we will explore why it is that suicide, depression, anxiety, and addiction are at all-time highs. The presence of depression, addiction, and anxiety are all correlated with excessive levels of resting cortisol. At the same time, consumerism seems to be playing a significant role in bringing about these states of chronic distress.

For the vast majority of our history as a civilization, people have owned very little. Possessions were held to a minimum as we only kept what was necessary for our survival. In the 18th century, when survival stopped being our primary concern, we began to acquire more esthetically pleasing objects. Purchases were no longer restricted to farming and hunting equipment but expanded to include clothing, cars, jewelry, and personal grooming. Esthetically attractive items weren't necessarily functional; some of them were quite impractical.

The Roman-Catholic church greatly criticized this cult of estheticism since it was, in their eyes, a cult of vanity, the father of the seven deadly sins. This shift to estheticism was criticized for the superficiality and hollowness it promoted. People became increasingly more interested in the way they looked than in the state their soul was in.

We don't need to be religious to understand that there's an issue with the values promoted by a consumerist economy. Tim Kasser is a social psychologist who has researched the effect that materialism has on mental health for the last 25 years. His findings are intuitive, but he used science to shine a discerning eye upon this subject.

The mechanism by which consumerism has increased depression, anxiety, and addiction in society is through promoting impulsivity and competitiveness. These

The Secrets To Improve Bloating, Digestion, Anxiety And Fat Loss

impulsive and competitive behaviors, in turn, are born from underlying extrinsic values that consumerism also stimulates (Kasser, 2018).

Meaning In Life & The Microbiome

First of all, we need to briefly define what values are. Values are our roadmap in life; they tell us when to go right or when to turn left. The reason values help us make decisions in life is because they're hierarchical in nature, meaning that we find some values more important than others. Perhaps you hold your value of freedom of expression over your value of financial security. Those values would make you discontent at a workplace that you feel oppresses your opinions.

We haven't always been as free to choose our path as we are today. In the dark medieval times, the church or the state would tell you what values are important and how you should live your life. This isn't the case anymore. We've been given a certain degree of freedom to choose what is important to us. With freedom comes responsibility though. Many people describe feeling lost, feeling like they have a void in their life. They have no sense of direction and a certain emptiness. In some regards, it must have been easier to be told what to do. The responsibility that comes with this newly acquired freedom means that we are the ones that must find our own path.

Consumerism is a step back in the evolution of people's journey to find meaning in their life. Its subtle control mechanisms strive to give you a purpose. Our economic system tells us that the benchmarks for success are having a "six-pack," buying the newest smartphone, having the largest home, having the most followers on social media networks, and taking a pill to feel better so you can buy more stuff.

The avoidance of pain and the search for pleasure is the purpose that society has programmed into us. When life has no meaning except for the pursuit of pleasure, life's struggles and difficulties can be quite difficult to face. The answer to every painful situation is simply to avoid the problem. If you feel sad, find a way of eliminating your sadness by going out and drinking. People, thus, go through great lengths to avoid their own darkness.

Instead of avoiding our darkness, we may try to understand it. We could see which underlying need of ours isn't being met. Perhaps our tendency to spend more time than we intend to on social media could really be seen as a warning sign telling us that we're lacking meaningful connections in our life. Perhaps, we're not spending enough time and energy to cultivate relationships that revitalize us through the sharing of common ground with others.

Getting a 9 to 5 job, marrying, having children, and taking out a home loan may be fulfilling for some, but it doesn't have to be everybody's purpose in life. Consequently, our values and the rewards we get from fulfilling these values should come from the inside; they should be intrinsic values chosen by us, not given to us.

One of the main issues with the extrinsic values promoted by our materialistic economic system is that it makes us base our sense of self-worth on others' opinions and possessions. When our self-esteem is based on a possession, it makes us susceptible to consumerism's mechanisms of envy and greed. You may argue and say I'm being pessimistic by calling our economic system greedy. You may say that what we're actually seeing is progress and a tendency towards constant improvement. I'm not against development, progress, and improvement. The issue is the continual dissatisfaction implied in greed and envy; those are the ugly sides of consumerism.

Constant dissatisfaction leaves absolutely no room for gratitude. In fact, constant dissatisfaction is what keeps us consuming. Genuinely fulfilling our needs is not good for business, just like curing a disease versus treating a disease is not as profitable. Is taking a supplement for the rest of your life truly necessary, or is that just what's good for business? Could we take a probiotic until our microbial biodiversity reaches a healthy equilibrium and then return to getting our microbes from a balanced diet? These are things I want you to ask yourself.

Our economic system looks to devalue your current possessions in order to motivate you to continue consuming. Let's say you fulfill your need to obtain the newest smartphone. Shortly after that, a new phone will be announced, but your sense of worth and status will take a blow if you don't acquire it. Then you may see your neighbor with the newer version, cave in and buy it. This is the mechanism of envy that consumerism uses. In this system, your possessions quickly become obsolete, fueling that desire inside to feel complete or whole. Again, they try to make you feel like you're not enough as you are.

On the other hand, when you strive to live your life by your own values, the rewards you strive for are internal. Financial security and health will naturally follow once you're on the right path. This isn't a mystical idea that I'm trying to convey to you. The act of feeling grateful actually reduces the amount of cortisol present in the body. As for following the right path, when you think you're on it, your brain will release dopamine, causing a reinforcing and pleasurable effect. So, there are hormonal processes that are involved in finding meaning in your life and not being mesmerized by materialistic values.

The right path is whatever you choose it to be. The path that is aligned with YOUR values. Not the ones imposed by your parents, religion, state, or media. This reward system has encouraged us to find our path or purpose all throughout evolutionary history. Our concerns are no longer solely about survival anymore. Our needs have evolved.

We now hold needs of a higher order such as safety, belonging, love and friendship, accomplishment, and realizing our true potential. An existential void is created when the gap between our current selves and our potential selves widens, as we begin to feel that we could have given the world so much more.

Depression and anxiety are natural consequences of a lack of meaning in our lives. The mechanisms by which depression, anxiety, and increased cortisol levels have to do with where we get our sense of self-worth, our outlook on life/society, and how we cope with life's struggles (how we deal with stress).

False values that are being sold to us as a road to happiness turn into coping mechanisms when we find out that they don't really fill the void inside us. Instead, they create a greater need for admiration, status, and power. This is similar to using salt in soft drinks to make people thirsty for more. Junk values are comparable to junk food in the sense that they do satisfy your needs for a while. However, if you continue to satisfy your need for food with burgers from McDonald's, it's going to take a toll on your body. The free radicals released through sugar, inflammation-causing pathogens, and the lack of nutrients per calorie will all have consequences. Consequences are a reduced amount of leptin, making you even hungrier, and becoming addicted to sugar and salt. When your need for food is satiated, though, it can even feel quite pleasurable to eat your favorite junk food.

In the same way, the pursuit of superficial materialistic purposes can be quite fulfilling in the moment. There are pleasurable activities like buying a new outfit impulsively or taking a selfie with the sole intention of getting attention and approval from others. At first, these activities are rewarding, but after some time, we begin to feel the void, the emptiness these pursuits bring.

This is why impulsivity is key to consumerism. Our economic system does not promote risk analysis or the delay of gratification. Consumerism makes us impulsive by telling us that life is all about fun and pleasure; it leaves no room for pain and discomfort. "If you feel bad, consume this! It'll make you feel better!" We're taught to drown out our worries and pains by consuming. It's a culture of numbing down the symptoms instead of addressing the root causes.

Impulsivity adds on to this ignorance. It makes us act instead of think. We simply consume without thinking about the consequences our actions may generate onto others or even our future selves. The act of not thinking about these consequences stimulates an individualistic, selfish way of living rooted in individualism and competition, rather than cooperation.

We have to ask ourselves, does this plan of continuous growth that our economic system proposes makes sense? Is it beneficial in the long run, or is it just a means to pursue pleasure in the present moment? Can our planet tolerate infinite growth, or are there limited resources?

If science did not support this view, I would not be talking to you about how materialistic values bring depression and anxiety through an existential emptiness. If this pursuit of selfish pleasure truly made people happy, I would not be making a case against it. Unfortunately, when we focus more of our time and energy on materialistic values, we end up with more depression, anxiety, and addiction (Kasser, 2018). We all have a combination of materialistic, superficial values, and intrinsic values. Mental health is correlated with leaning more towards the intrinsic values.

The correlations are clear between superficial, materialistic, and selfish behavior and higher levels of mental distress. The mechanisms by which this happens is a topic for a whole other day. This problem concerns us as far as cortisol levels and inflammation goes, so finding a true purpose and questioning your values, in the end, are also tied into our gut health.

I can't give you a purpose. Nobody can. That's something you must find on your own. Finding your path is just as important as eating the right foods. The emptiness you can feel from using somebody else's formula for happiness will leave you with a sense of meaninglessness. If you have no purpose, why would you get up in the morning and go to work? Simple tasks, such as going to work, become so painful and stressful that we can become overwhelmed.

Have you ever asked yourself why you want to be healthy? Why is it that you're doing the things you're doing in your life? Why are you reading this book? Some people go to school, get a job, and get married without even asking themselves if that's what they really wanted in life. When you ask them, they might say, "well, that's just what everybody else does."

What are your values? Can you make a list of at least ten values you hold? Ask yourself whether the life you're living is truly aligned with those ten values.

Consumerism preys on our insecurities by telling us we're not enough. The discourse is that we will be whole once we acquire the product that is being sold to us. Could this be happening in the health and supplement industries as well? Could they be taking advantage of the fact that we want to be healthy, and could they be telling us that we need their product to be whole?

I would like for you to question these possibilities whenever you're reading about the next biggest hype when it comes to healthy lifestyle products.

The energy we spend trying to acquire a product is the energy that could be put into working on our health. By delaying our gratification, by leaning into discomfort, we are actually taking ourselves back.

What We Know About the Microbiome

Media, such as magazines, videos, and news feeds make it sound that they know exactly how the microbiome works. As we've reviewed, these metabolic processes are quite complex. We've only scratched the surface of an extremely complex subject. A subject that's very interesting and research in this area holds great promise. This scientific research field is in its infancy, so we should be wary of being swept off our feet by propaganda.

We now know that we can't rely on a single microorganism as a cure-all, since all our microbiomes are different. Depending on what kind of environment we create, our microorganisms may serve us well or work against us. This is why advertising a single strain as the cure-all option can be misleading.

No matter how many probiotics you pump into your body, if you're not dealing with the stress in your life adequately, sleep well, and eat well, you're not going to get the results that are promised to you. Restrictive diets may not be the solution for every individual. These diets could even decrease your microbial biodiversity by making fewer nutrients available in your microbiome.

We simply don't know how to heal our gut yet. We don't have a fail-proof step-by-step guide for everybody to apply. The findings we have from experimental research aren't always conclusive. The ones done on animals help but don't fully translate to us, and even the ones done on humans have conflicting results. All this means is that we lack a great deal of understanding on the subject.

What we do know is that inflammation is correlated with less microbial biodiversity. Our microbial biodiversity is affected by excess levels of stress or insulin. Cortisol increases our resistance to insulin, increasing how much insulin is present in our body and leading to further inflammation. Inflammation in our gut loosens the tight junctions of our intestinal wall leading to a leaky gut. Our gut leaks inflammation-causing molecules throughout our body only to cause damage and inflammation throughout the rest of our body. This may explain one of the reasons that gastrointestinal diseases are correlated with mental health. Our mental states and our outlook on life influence how we deal with life's struggles and the way we deal with stress. Stress is correlated with high levels of cortisol, which gives us one of the main clues as to how to deal with gut health.

Increasing the amount of fiber-rich foods and decreasing the amount of refined sugars you consume is a simple practice that we should all be following. Less than 25 grams of sugar and more than 30 grams of fiber daily is key to microbial biodiversity. Colorful fruit, healthy fats, and fermented foods can all act as probiotics, prebiotics, and antioxidants.

Exercising and finding ways to reduce cortisol accumulation in the body is essential to our health for many reasons, not just for our gut health. Health comes from a root word that means "whole," which in itself should tell you how we should be treating our body. We should be treating it as a whole complex system with many parts that interact with each other. Instead of targeting one area of our body, we should be targeting our general wellbeing.

Even our body doesn't exist isolated. We're part of a whole system ourselves, part of an ecosystem, part of a society. The effects our social environment has on our health are profound, and we should be aware of how society impacts our outlook on our lives. Things that are seemingly unrelated, like having a purpose in your life, and the state of your microbial biodiversity, may very well have extensive connections with each other.

There is much work to be done, and in the end, it's just that, work. There are no cutting corners. Becoming self-aware and making conscious decisions about how we treat ourselves and our environment is crucial to our wellbeing. The first step, that you have taken already, is you've become aware. Now it's time for you to commit to changing your life. Values and ideals are only potentialities until we commit to them through our actions.

How are you going to spend the next months of your life? Are you going to fit more meaningful and enriching activities into your life? The energy spent on finding products to heal yourself can be spent into activities that you already know heal you. I understand there's a lot of conflicting information about how we should eat and what is healthy and what is not. The only way to know if it works for you is through experience. Also, your experience is just that, your own.

If evidence is found for a fail-proof method for long-lasting health or ever-lasting beauty, trust me, I'm going to tell you about it. I'm always keeping up to date with the newest scientific research, and I am eager to research more.

Final Words

Pain, suffering, and disease are inevitable parts of life, just like death is inseparable from life. We've tried to intervene in these processes by eliminating anything that causes us suffering. Since ancient times we've been looking for something to blame for all our misfortunes and diseases. We've gone from blaming ethereal entities to microscopic beings.

We've discussed what a microbiome is, and we have described the competitive scenario our microbiota live in and what our role is as far as how we tilt the scale of the microbial war in our favor. After all, it's in our best interest to help our microbiota thrive and propagate in a balanced manner.

Imbalances can arise from not having enough microorganisms to colonize us. Perhaps our environment was too clean, and we were not exposed to microbes, or maybe our diet was too restrictive. Dysbiosis can also occur from not giving our microbiota what they want. Even our good bacteria can turn pathogenic when they're forced to switch food sources. Not enough fiber will force some organisms to switch to sugar and possibly turn them into pathobionts.

Imbalances can occur in many ways, but one thing most of them have in common is that they lead to inflammation. Inflammation in our intestinal lining is due to bacterial overgrowths or the productions of corrosive metabolites. Chronic inflammation makes our gut leak toxins into our bloodstream. They are then transported to our brain's glial cells, muscles, joints, and even other organs.

The toxins floating around in our body are thought to be one of the leading reasons that IBS coexists with mental health and autoimmune diseases. These toxins over excite our immune system and turn our defenses against us, making our inflammation damage the very cells it was supposed to protect.

The overgrowth of our colonic bacteria that spills over into our small intestine seems to be caused by an imbalance in the sugar to fiber ratio found in our diet. SIBO causes a decrease in some of our commensal bacteria that are involved in the production of hormones necessary for regulating our body weight. Our body can be strongly affected by this hormonal imbalance, but this is not a moral failing. Eating enough fiber to stay satiated longer and prevent a SIBO is essential to control how our body stores fat.

Probiotics are important for maintaining equilibrium in our body. However, we're

The Secrets To Improve Bloating, Digestion, Anxiety And Fat Loss

not sure how many of which organisms each person needs to take. To be able to prescribe probiotics, the responsible thing to do would be to genetically sequence your microbiome, while checking your hormonal equilibrium. For the time being, we should look to get most of our probiotics from a balanced diet, just like we always have.

Our stress levels seem to interact directly with our microbiome's diversity and even our body's insulin resistance. Stress can be caused by our minds or by real situations, but that really doesn't matter. Our body treats both the same way. Prolonged periods of stress and the inability to burn the energy that stress makes available leads to increased resistance to insulin. Cortisol, the stress hormone, is responsible for making energy available and spending it, while insulin is responsible for storing the energy in our body for later use.

Increased levels of resting cortisol seem to be a key factor in dysbiosis and mental health disorders. We're unsure if cortisol is a cause or effect when it comes to these disorders, but it's most likely both. Cortisol tips the scale for pathogens that compete with the commensal bacteria that produce serotonin and dopamine. Consequently, higher cortisol levels mean lower levels of serotonin and dopamine because of the dysbiosis that is being caused. Dysbiosis through chronic stress seems to be a potential cause for anxiety and depression.

Regulating our stress levels and getting enough sleep is essential for our gut, mind, and overall health. Sleep is regulated by biorhythms that modulate our cortisol and melatonin levels. Cortisol is released to get us active and going, while melatonin helps us unwind at night. Cortisol suppresses sleep, and melatonin suppresses production. Learning to relax and creating proper bedtime habits are crucial to our hormonal equilibrium.

It's great if you're watching what you eat, how much you eat, and when you eat. Let's say you even incorporate exercising, but if you're not sleeping well, you're pretty much swimming upstream. Maintaining your body processes efficiently and healthily requires a holistic approach. Finding this path is part of this holistic approach. Feeling like your life is meaningless or adopting false ideals as your road to happiness will only disrupt the hormonal processes you're working so hard to tame.

Understanding your place in society and our economic system's goals is imperative to your gut health. I'm sure that, before you read through this work, you had never associated your gut health with finding a purpose in life. Living solely to consume and seek pleasure is correlated with depression and anxiety, and we know that these disorders lead to increased levels of stress. We're not isolated beings.

We're part of a system, part of a society, and part of a planet.

Just like the microbiome that makes us who we are, so too does the biome make the planet what it is. We're part of the biome, and we can decide if we want to be treated like a pathogenic disease that needs to be eliminated or if we want to be more like our commensal bacteria and make this world a better place.

References

Alcock J, Maley CC, Aktipis CA. Is eating behavior manipulated by the gastrointestinal microbiota? Evolutionary pressures and potential mechanisms. Bioessays. 2014 Oct;36(10):940-9. doi: 10.1002/bies.201400071. Epub 2014 Aug 8. PMID: 25103109; PMCID: PMC4270213.

Allaband, C., McDonald, D., Vázquez-Baeza, Y., Minich, J. J., Tripathi, A., Brenner, D. A., Loomba, R., Smarr, L., Sandborn, W. J., Schnabl, B., Dorrestein, P., Zarrinpar, A., & Knight, R. (2019). Microbiome 101: Studying, Analyzing, and Interpreting Gut Microbiome Data for Clinicians. Clinical gastroenterology and hepatology : the official clinical practice journal of the American Gastroenterological Association, 17(2), 218–230. https://doi.org/10.1016/j.cgh.2018.09.017

Aristotle. (1925). Nichomachean ethics: Book II. (W.D. Ross, Trans.). Retrieved from The Internet Classics Archive: http://classics.mit.edu (Original work published 350 B.C.E)

BallenaBlanca / CC BY-SA (https://creativecommons.org/licenses/by-sa/4.0)

Belkaid, Y., & Hand, T. W. (2014). Role of the microbiota in immunity and inflammation. Cell, 157(1), 121–141. https://doi.org/10.1016/j.cell.2014.03.011

Benedé, S., Blázquez, A. B., Chiang, D., Tordesillas, L., & Berin, M. C. (2016). The rise of food allergy: Environmental factors and emerging treatments. EBioMedicine, 7, 27-34. https://doi.org/10.1016/j.ebiom.2016.04.012

Bloomfield, S. F., Rook, G. A., Scott, E. A., Shanahan, F., Stanwell-Smith, R., & Turner, P. (2016). Time to abandon the hygiene hypothesis: New perspectives on allergic disease, the human microbiome, infectious disease prevention and the role of targeted hygiene. Perspectives in Public Health, 136(4), 213-224. https://doi.org/10.1177/1757913916650225

Canavan C, West J, Card T. The epidemiology of irritable bowel syndrome. Clin Epidemiol. 2014 Feb 4;6:71-80. doi: 10.2147/CLEP.S40245. PMID: 24523597; PMCID: PMC3921083.

Cani P., Human gut microbiome: hopes, threats and promises Gut 2 018;67:1716-1725.

Cardenas, Diana. (2013). Let not thy food be confused with thy medicine: The Hippocratic misquotation. e-SPEN the European e-Journal of Clinical Nutrition and Metabolism. XXX. 10.1016/j.clnme.2013.10.002.

Chassaing, B., Van de Wiele, T., De Bodt, J., Marzorati, M., & Gewirtz, A. T. (2017). Dietary emulsifiers directly alter human microbiota composition and gene expression ex vivo potentiating intestinal inflammation. Gut, 66(8), 1414–1427. https://doi.org/10.1136/gutjnl-2016-313099

Cohen H. (1953). The Evolution of the Concept of Disease. Proceedings of the Royal Society of Medicine , 48(155), 2-6.

Dunn AB, Jordan S, Baker BJ, Carlson NS. The Maternal Infant Microbiome: Considerations for Labor and Birth. MCN Am J Matern Child Nurs. 2017 Nov/Dec;42(6):318-325. doi: 10.1097/NMC.0000000000000373. PMID: 28825919; PMCID: PMC5648605.

Ebneshsahidi. (2006). The Digestive System. Benjamin Cummings.

Fung, J. (2016). The obesity code: Unlocking the secrets of weight loss. Greystone Books.

Jane A. Foster, Linda Rinaman, L. I., & John F. Cryan, J. O. (2017). Stress & the gut-brain axis: Regulation by the microbiome. Neurobiology of Stress, 7, 124-136. https://doi.org/10.1016/j.ynstr.2017.03.001

The Secrets To Improve Bloating, Digestion, Anxiety And Fat Loss

García, Apolinaria & Navarro, Karen & Sanhueza Carrera, Enrique & Pineda, Susana & Pastene, Edgar & Quezada, Marilyn & Henríquez, Karem & Karlyshev, Andrey & Villena, Julio & González, Carlos. (2016). Characterization of Lactobacillus fermentum UCO-979C, a probiotic strain with a potent anti-Helicobacter pylori activity. Electronic Journal of Biotechnology. 25. 10.1016/j.ejbt.2016.11.008.

Kasser, Tim & Ahuvia, Aaron. (2002). Materialistic Values and Well-Being in Business Students. European Journal of Social Psychology. 32. 137 - 146. 10.1002/ejsp.85.

Khan, M. F., & Wang, H. (2020). Environmental exposures and autoimmune diseases: Contribution of gut microbiome. Frontiers in Immunology, 10. https://doi.org/10.3389/fimmu.2019.03094

Massarrat S, Saniee P, Siavoshi F, Mokhtari R, Mansour-Ghanaei F, Khalili-Samani S. The Effect of Helicobacter pylori Infection, Aging, and Consumption of Proton Pump Inhibitor on Fungal Colonization in the Stomach of Dyspeptic Patients. Front Microbiol. 2016 May 25;7:801. doi: 10.3389/fmicb.2016.00801. PMID: 27252698; PMCID: PMC4879133.

Mattson, M., Moehl, K., Ghena, N. et al. Intermittent metabolic switching, neuroplasticity and brain health. Nat Rev Neurosci 19, 81–94 (2018). https://doi.org/10.1038/nrn.2017.156

Mawdsley, J. E., & Rampton, D. S. (2005). Psychological stress in IBD: new insights into pathogenic and therapeutic implications. Gut, 5 4(10), 1481–1491. https://doi.org/10.1136/gut.2005.064261

Mayer, E. A., Padua, D., & Tillisch, K. (2014). Altered brain-gut axis in autism: Cormobidity or causative mechanisms? BioEssays, 36(10), 933-939. https://doi.org/10.1002/bies.201400075

Misra, Snigdha & Mohanty, Debapriya. (2017). Psychobiotics: A new approach for treating mental illness?. Critical Reviews in Food Science and Nutrition. 59. 1-7. 10.1080/10408398.2017.1399860.

Lewis SJ, Heaton KW (1997) Stool form scale as a useful guide to intestinal transit time. Scandinavian Jorunal of Gastroenterology 32: 920–4

Li, Y., Hao, Y., Fan, F., & Zhang, B. (2018). The Role of Microbiome in Insomnia, Circadian Disturbance and Depression. Frontiers in psychiatry, 9 , 669. https://doi.org/10.3389/fpsyt.2018.00669

Payne, J. D., & Nadel, L. (2004). Sleep, dreams, and memory consolidation: the role of the stress hormone cortisol . Tucson, AZ: Cold Spring Harbor Laboratory Press.

Prescott, Susan. (2017). History of Medicine: Origin of the Term Microbiome and why it Matters. Human Microbiome Journal. 4. 10.1016/j.humic.2017.05.004.

Rogers, G. B., Keating, D. J., Young, R. L., Wong, M. L., Licinio, J., and Wesselingh, S. (2016). From gut dysbiosis to altered brain function and mental illness: mechanisms and pathways. Mol. Psychiatry 21, 738–748. doi: 10.1038/mp.2016.50

Sharon, G., Sampson, T. R., Geschwind, D. H., & Mazmanian, S. K. (2016). The Central Nervous System and the Gut Microbiome. Cell, 167(4), 915–932. https://doi.org/10.1016/j.cell.2016.10.027

Rienzi, Robert A Britton, Adaptation of the Gut Microbiota to Modern Dietary Sugars and Sweeteners, Advances in Nutrition, Volume 11, Issue 3, May 2020, Pages 616–629, https://doi.org/10.1093/advances/nmz118

Ludzki, Leszek & Maes, Michael. (2020). From "leaky gut" to impaired glia-neuron communication in depression. 10.13140/RG.2.2.18845.74720.

SAMHSA. (2014). Treating Sleep Problems of People in Recovery From Substance Use Disorders. In Brief, 8(2).

Sanmiguel C, Gupta A, Mayer EA. Gut Microbiome and Obesity: A Plausible Explanation for Obesity. Curr Obes Rep. 2015 Jun;4(2):250-61. doi: 10.1007/s13679-015-0152-0. PMID: 26029487; PMCID: PMC4443745.

Segovia, F. J., Hidalgo, G. I., Villasante, J., Ramis, X., & Almajano, M. P. (2018). Avocado Seed: A Comparative Study of Antioxidant Content and Capacity in Protecting Oil Models from Oxidation. Molecules (Basel, Switzerland), 23(10), 2421. https://doi.org/10.3390/molecules23102421

Shumsky, N. (1998). Encyclopedia of Urban America: The Cities and Suburbs (Volume 1 ed.) NY: ABC-CLIO.

Singh, R.K., Chang, H., Yan, D. e t al. Influence of diet on the gut microbiome and implications for human health. J Transl Med 15, 73 (2017). https://doi.org/10.1186/s12967-017-1175-y

Spector, Tim & Gardner, Christopher. (2020). Challenges and opportunities for better nutrition science—an essay by Tim Spector and Christopher Gardner. BMJ. 369. m2470. 10.1136/bmj.m2470.

Stossel, S. (2014). My age of anxiety: Fear, hope, dread, and the search for peace of mind. Vintage.

Thantsha, Mapitsi & Mamvura Mbiriri, Chiedza & Booyens, J.. (2012). Probiotics - What They Are, Their Benefits and Challenges. 10.5772/32889.

Vivekanudeep, Karri & Hirschi, Kendal. (2020). Gut Bacteria have a novel sweet tooth: ribose sensing and scavenging from fiber. Gut Microbes. 11. 1-3. 10.1080/19490976.2020.1770667.

Zanetti, Ana & Rogero, Marcelo & Atzingen, Maria. (2018). Low-FODMAP diet in the management of irritable bowel syndrome. Nutrire. 43. 10.1186/s41110-018-0076-z.

Zhong, Yan & Priebe, Marion & Vonk, Roel & Huang, Cheng-Yu & Antoine, Jean-Michel & He, Tao & Harmsen, Hermie & Welling, Gjalt. (2004). The Role of Colonic Microbiota in Lactose Intolerance. Digestive diseases and sciences. 49. 78-83. 10.1023/B:DDAS.0000011606.96795.40.

Zuo, T., & Ng, S. C. (2018). The gut microbiota in the pathogenesis and therapeutics of inflammatory bowel disease. Frontiers in Microbiology, 9. https://doi.org/10.3389/fmicb.2018.02247

The Secrets To Improve Bloating, Digestion,
Anxiety And Fat Loss

Milton Keynes UK
Ingram Content Group UK Ltd.
UKHW050943020823
426115UK00030B/155

9 781953 142313